# NUT

## AN INT

# WENDY DOYLE

Hodder & Stoughton

A MEMBER OF THE HODDER HEADLINE GROUP

## Acknowledgements

I would like to thank Professor Michael Crawford and all my colleagues at the Institute of Brain Chemistry and Human Nutrition for their help and support in writing this book. I would also like to express my appreciation to Maggie Sanderson, Barbara Flowerdew and other friends who gave me so much encouragement.

*British Library Cataloguing in Publication Data*

ISBN 0-340-64398-6

First published 1994 as *Teach Yourself Healthy Eating*
Re-published 1995 as *Nutrition: An Introduction*
Impression number    10 9 8 7 6 5 4 3 2
Year                          1999   1998   1997   1996

Typeset by Rowland Phototypesetting Ltd, Bury St Edmunds, Suffolk.
Printed in Great Britain for Hodder & Stoughton Educational,
a division of Hodder Headline Plc, 338 Euston Road, London NW1 3BH
by Cox & Wyman Ltd, Reading, Berks.

# — CONTENTS —

# —— INTRODUCTION ——

## —— Introduction to nutrition ——

> It's a very odd thing,
> As odd as can be
> That whatever Miss T eats
> Turns into Miss T.
>
> *Walter de la Mare*

Whether you want to live to be 100 or would rather settle for threescore years and ten, it is important to us all to look good and feel well. Food can be such a pleasurable part of our lives that it is easy to forget that it also ensures our survival through the nourishment it provides. We concern ourselves with food several times a day, and there is no practice that influences our health more than the choice and amount of food we eat. The body is the product of what it eats in much the same way as a cake is the product of the ingredients from which it is made – we are what we eat.

The first principle of healthy eating is that requirements of all essential nutrients are met. Most people in developed countries are now generally considered to be 'well fed', with little evidence of malnutrition. However, malnutrition is not peculiar to Third World countries. It occurs whenever the body is not adequately served by the food it eats. Although often associated with undernutrition, it can equally mean overeating, particularly when associated with imbalances such as too much fat or too much sugar in your diet.

For most of human experience, as hunter-gatherers, people ate fruit, berries, nuts, seeds, roots and leaves. They caught fish and hunted game but, for the most part, they ate much more food of vegetable origin and less of animal products. This was the diet with which the human race evolved and it was the diet that the human body was biochemically designed to handle.

Today, radical changes in methods of food production, processing and marketing have caused food habits to move away from our evolutionary diet. Supermarket shelves are laden with an enormous array of foods to choose from; it is easy to succumb to the highly skilled marketing techniques which tempt us away from the foods of nature and towards the attractively packaged, highly processed foods. These factory foods no longer retain their natural complement of fibre, vitamins and minerals. With these changes have come imbalances in the nutritional composition of our diets, characterised by an excess of calorie-dense foods of low nutritional value. Fat and refined sugar now account for over half our energy intake, yet other than fat-soluble vitamins and essential fatty acids, they provide no protein, minerals or water-soluble vitamins. That means we have to rely on less than half our calories to meet our requirements for these nutrients which are so essential to health.

Fifty years ago, public health problems were associated with interrelated problems of lower resistance to infections, often fatal infectious diseases such as tuberculosis and dietary deficiencies such as rickets. Today, the major causes of death have shifted from infectious to chronic degenerative diseases, such as heart disease and cancer, many of which are nutrition related. The remarkable increase in some chronic diseases over the last 35–40 years has increased the pressure on governments to encourage preventive policies to these diseases. In the UK alone, millions of people are suffering from diseases that could have been prevented. Every year, thousands of lives are wasted by premature suffering and death from disease caused, at least in part, by the food we eat.

It is important, therefore, that we should all be in a position to make informed decisions about our choice of food. What I hope this book will do is to remove some of the mystique about healthy eating and to provide you with facts on which to base your judgement when planning your menus or making purchasing decisions, faced, for instance, with a choice of 20 different margarines in the supermarket.

You don't have to give up everything you love to protect your health. Healthy eating is not incompatible with pleasurable eating – it is not a list of don'ts. It is one of the most positive things you can do for your own health and well-being. Remember, food is for enjoying, and the aim of this book is not to leave you feeling guilt-ridden about what you eat, but to inform and encourage you to understand the principles of good nutrition and make sensible decisions about your own everyday diet.

# 1

# FOOD COMPOSITION

Because eating is such a pleasurable activity, we tend to overlook the fact that the foods we eat are used to sustain life. Food maintains and builds body tissues, regulates body processes and supplies the body with heat or other forms of energy. Food is made up of protein, fat, carbohydrate, water, vitamins and minerals. A chemical analysis of a food such as cabbage would show that it contained many different nutrients but that the main component was water (90 per cent). The remaining solid matter is made up of carbohydrate, protein, fat, vitamins and minerals (see table below).

| component | % | |
|-----------|------|---|
| water | 90.0 | |
| protein | 1.7 | |
| carbohydrate | 4.1 | |
| fat | 0.4 | |
| vitamins | 0.1 | (carotene, vitamin E, thiamin, riboflavin, niacin, pyridoxine, folate, panothenic acid, biotin, vitamin C) |
| minerals | 0.4 | (sodium, potassium, calcium, magnesium, phosphorus, iron, copper, zinc, chloride, manganese, selenium, iodine) |

An analysis of cabbage

Carbohydrates, protein and fat are the three main sources of energy in our diet. These 'macronutrients' are present in the food we eat in relatively large amounts. Protein is made up of about 20 amino acids, of which eight are essential for growth and normal functioning of the body.

Similarly, fat is made up of over 40 fatty acids, only two of which are thought to be essential to adult health. Carbohydrates include sugars, starches and fibre or non-starch polysaccharides. Alcohol also contributes to energy intake. The average man in the UK consumes 272g of carbohydrate, 85g of protein, 102g of fat and 25g of alcohol every day, providing him with 2,450 kilocalories.

The micronutrients, i.e. vitamins, minerals and trace elements, are present in only small amounts. Most foods contain a variety of nutrients but all foods are low in one, and usually more, essential nutrients, so your requirements are only likely to be met if a variety of foods are eaten. Scientists have identified 16 different vitamins and 20 minerals which are essential to human health.

Not all components of food provide us with energy or nutrients, and not all components are essential to life. For example, insoluble fibre, now more commonly called non-starch polysaccharides (NSP), is not absorbed from the gut and so is not considered a nutrient; however, while not being essential to life, fibre is associated with health because of its role in the correct functioning of the bowel, and its absence from the diet may increase the risk of bowel disease.

Most foods contain significant amounts of water. Water does not provide calories and so the more water a food contains, the lower its energy content; for instance, 96 per cent of the weight of a cucumber is water and it contains only 10 kilocalories in 100g (3.5oz) of cucumber. In contrast, sugar contains only a trace of water and provides 394 kilocalories in 100g. Water from food can contribute about half the body's daily water needs.

# Energy

The ultimate source of all energy in living organisms is the sun. Plants transform heat and light (a process known as 'photosynthesis') into energy, which is stored as potential energy within different plant foods. Animals, including man, are unable to use energy directly from the sun and so rely on energy from plant sources.

To find out how many kilocalories a food provides, a laboratory scientist can burn the food in a chamber called a 'bomb calorimeter', used to measure heat production. Over 200 years ago, a French scientist called

Lavoisier showed that food supplies energy to the body in similar amounts that would be produced as heat by burning the food.

Energy has traditionally been expressed as kilocalories. By definition, one Calorie is the amount of heat required to raise 1kg (2.2lb) of water by 1°C. The Calorie with a capital C is the same as the kilocalorie, which is 1,000 calories.

## New terminology

More recently, in line with the International Organisation for Standardisation, the preferred units of energy have been changed to the 'kilojoule' (kJ). To convert kilocalories to kilojoules, multiply kilocalories by 4.184 (or approximate by using 4.2). So, someone having 2,500 kilocalories a day would be having approximately 10,000 kilojoules (10,460) or 10 megajoules.

## Energy value of food

When food is burned up (oxidised) by the body, 1g of protein provides approximately 4 kilocalories; 1g of carbohydrate, 3.75 kilocalories; 1g of fat, 9 kilocalories; 1g of alcohol (ethanol), 7 kilocalories. So, if you know the protein, fat and carbohydrate content of a food, you can work out the calorie or energy content. Let's take milk as an example:

**Milk (full fat)**

|  | grams per 100g (3.5oz) of milk |  | kcals per gram |  | kcals per 100g | % of energy from |
|---|---|---|---|---|---|---|
| Carbohydrate | 4.8 | × | 3.75 | = | 18.0 | 27.3% |
| Protein | 3.2 | × | 4 | = | 12.8 | 19.4% |
| Fat | 3.9 | × | 9 | = | 35.1 | 53.3% |
| Water | 87.8 | × | 0 | = | 0.0 |  |
|  | 99.7 |  |  |  | 65.9 |  |

This table shows that, weight for weight, fat is the most energy-dense nutrient (9 kcals/gram), with more than 50 per cent of the kilocalories being derived from fat.

So, 100g of whole milk contains approximately 66 kilocalories or 375 kilocalories in a pint (567g):

$$1 \text{ pint milk (567ml)} = \frac{567 \times 66}{100} = 375 \text{ kcals}$$

## *Energy requirements*

Just as a car needs fuel to work, so too does your body. It doesn't matter whether the action is voluntary, such as walking, or involuntary, such as maintaining muscle tone, digestion of food or transmission of nerve impulses. If more energy is required for these functions than is provided for by the intake of food, energy reserves, fat stored in the body (adipose tissue), will be used up. By the same principle, any excess energy provided by too much food will be stored in the body as fat, which will act as an energy reserve. When energy intake equals energy expenditure, equilibrium results and body weight is maintained, regardless of whether you are above, below or within the normal weight range for your height.

Energy requirements have to take five factors into consideration: size and sex of an individual, their energy expenditure, any special needs such as pregnancy and growth, and their basal metabolic rate. Basal metabolic rate (BMR) is simply the rate at which the body uses energy when at complete rest. This will include energy to maintain body temperature and other normal functions such as breathing, pumping blood from the heart and other involuntary activities like brain function. In adults, the metabolic rate is proportional to the amount of lean body tissue, so women tend to have lower basal metabolic rates than men because they are lighter and have a higher fat-to-lean ratio. The average daily energy requirement for an adult woman is 1,940 kilocalories (8.1 kilojoules) and for a man is 2,550 kilocalories (10.6 kilojoules). In contrast, it is estimated that a male elephant, carrying out strenuous work, requires around 92,000 kilocalories a day, while a moderately active canary requires 11 kilocalories a day!

Other foods 4%

Egg & egg dishes 2%

Fish & fish dishes 2%

Fruit & nuts 2%

Sugar, confectionery & preserves 8%

Fat spread 6%

*of which:*
Bread 13%
Biscuits, cakes & buns 9%

Cereal & cereal products 8%

Beverages 9%

Meat & meat products 16%

Milk & milk products 11%

Vegetables 12%

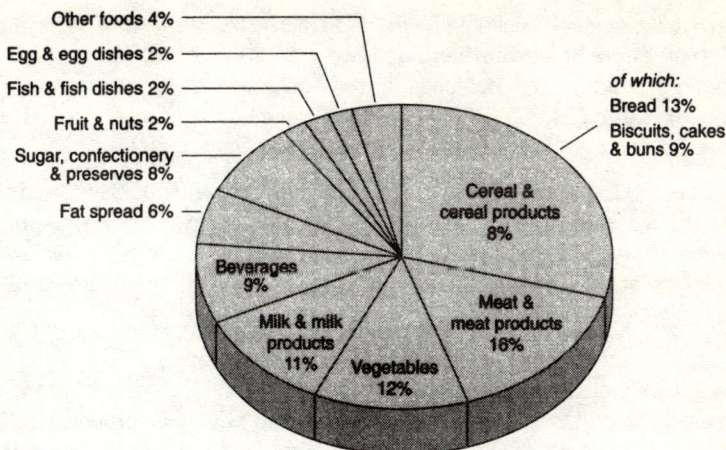

Sources of energy in the UK diet (British Adult Survey, 1990)

# Fat

Fat makes food taste better, it contributes to the flavour and improves the texture of food. It also helps to satisfy the appetite and, because fat is digested from the stomach more slowly than other nutrients, it helps to delay the return of hunger.

Fat is a concentrated source of energy, supplying 9 kilocalories per gram – more than twice the amount supplied by carbohydrate or protein on a weight-for-weight basis. Besides being a source of energy, dietary fats have other important functions. They provide transport and help the body to absorb the fat-soluble vitamins (A, D, E and K). Some body fat is essential as it cushions and protects organs such as the liver and kidneys and it also helps to insulate and keep us warm. Certain fats are essential to health and are often referred to as the 'essential fatty acids'. This is because they are a vital component of all cell structures, but they cannot be manufactured by the body and so have to be obtained from food.

## Different types of fats

The basic building blocks of fat are fatty acids. Over 40 different fatty acids occur in nature, of which about 21 are found in significant amounts in an average diet. Depending on their chemical structure, fatty acids may be saturated or unsaturated. If they are unsaturated, they may be monounsaturated or polyunsaturated. Whether they are saturated, monounsaturated or polyunsaturated makes no difference to their energy value, which is 9 kilocalories in every gram of fat.

A fat or oil can often be referred to as a saturated fat, a monounsaturated fat or a polyunsaturated fat, depending on which group of fatty acids they contain most of. This is not strictly true, because no food or oil contains just one type of fatty acid; instead they are made up of a mixture of fatty acids.

One of the most important differences in fatty acid properties is illustrated by how hard or liquid a fat or oil is. For example, butter and lard, which are animal fats and are predominantly saturated, are solid at room temperature. On the other hand, olive oil, which is predominantly monounsaturated, will be 'mushy' or cloudy if kept in a fridge but liquid in a warm atmosphere; sunflower oil, predominantly polyunsaturated, will always be liquid at room temperature. Cold-water fish contain a high proportion of polyunsaturates – if they contained lots of saturated fats they would seize up and become solid in cold waters!

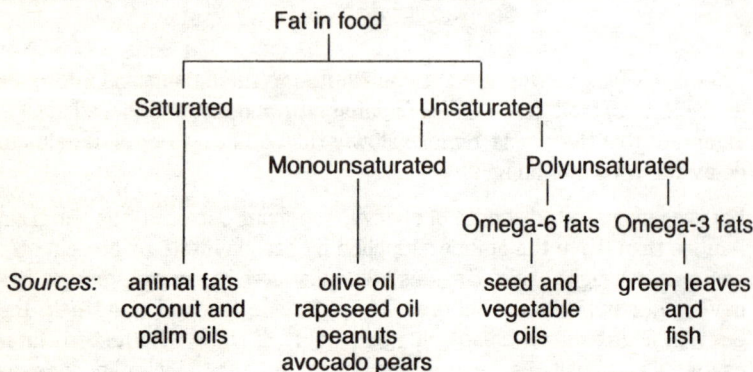

```
                          Fat in food
          ┌───────────────────┴───────────────────┐
      Saturated                              Unsaturated
          │                      ┌────────────────┴────────┐
          │                Monounsaturated           Polyunsaturated
          │                      │                ┌─────────┴─────────┐
          │                      │           Omega-6 fats     Omega-3 fats
          │                      │                │                │
Sources:  animal fats        olive oil       seed and       green leaves
          coconut and        rapeseed oil    vegetable          and
          palm oils          peanuts         oils              fish
                             avocado pears
```

Different fats in food

|  | Saturated fat | Monounsaturated fat | Polyunsaturated fat | |
|---|---|---|---|---|
|  |  |  | omega-6 | omega-3 |
| By men: | 42.0 | 31.4 | 13.8 | 1.83 |
| By women: | 31.1 | 22.1 | 9.6 | 1.35 |

Average amount of fat eaten, in grams per day (British Adult Survey, 1990)

## Saturated fats

Eating too much saturated fat is linked with raised blood cholesterol levels and hence with increased risk of heart disease, the most common cause of death in the UK.

Animal fats, such as fat on meat, lard and dripping, cream, milk and cheese, all contain a high proportion of saturated fat. Coconut and palm oils are also rich in saturated fat, so do not be lulled into believing that all vegetable fats and oils are healthy. Coconut and palm oils are often used in commercially prepared cakes and biscuits because saturated fats are chemically more stable than unsaturated fats and have a long shelf life. Their use minimises the formation of rancid flavours in food during storage, which has an obvious value to food manufacturers.

## Monounsaturated fats

Monounsaturated fats have been considered to be neutral as far as health is concerned – not thought to be 'good' or 'bad' for health. However, Greece and other Mediterranean countries, where consumption of olive oil is high, have very low rates of heart disease. This may, of course, be partly attributed to their lower intake of saturated fat and their higher intake of fruit and vegetables but, nevertheless, monounsaturates are now generally considered to have a protective effect against heart disease. Olive oil, rapeseed oil, avocado pears and peanuts are all good sources of monounsaturates.

## Polyunsaturated fats

Polyunsaturated fatty acids are thought to promote a healthy circulation and therefore be beneficial to health. Our body can make saturated fat from carbohydrate and from some proteins when there is more energy in the diet than is required. We are also able to convert saturated fat into monounsaturated fat. However, we are unable to make some polyunsaturated fatty acids which are essential components of all cell membranes and must, therefore, be obtained directly from the food we eat. These polyunsaturated fatty acids are often referred to as 'essential fatty acids' (EFAs). Polyunsaturated fats are found mainly in vegetable and seed oils and their margarines, oily fish and lean meat.

## Two families of EFAs

There are two principal families of EFAs: the omega-6 family and the omega-3 family. The nutritional significance of these two families has really only been understood since the late 1970s and much research is still being done on the health effects of each family.

Most Western-type diets contain about ten times as many omega-6 fatty acids to omega-3, and the omega-6 family were generally thought to be of more importance nutritionally. However, in 1978 it was observed that Eskimos living in their own environment, eating large quantities of fish and other marine foods high in omega-3 fatty acids, did not suffer from heart disease, but when they moved to live in Denmark and ate Western-type foods, they suffered the same circulatory problems as the Danes. Since then, the omega-3 family has been shown to play a role, not just in prevention of heart disease but in slowing certain types of tumour growth and inflammatory diseases such as psoriasis and rheumatoid arthritis.

The EFAs have two major functions. First, they play important structural roles in cell membranes. The second major function is regulatory: they are involved in the regulation of immune and other functions such as blood clotting, hence the extended bleeding time reported in Eskimos consuming a diet high in fish and marine foods.

## Food sources of EFAs

**Lean meat:** lean muscle tissue contains both omega-6 and omega-3 families.

**Seed oils:** contain mainly omega-6 fatty acids. Seed and nut oils such as sunflower, corn and soya, and margarines made from these, are mostly good sources of omega-6 fatty acids. Two exceptions, in that they contain appreciable amounts of both families, are soyabean oil (about 50 per cent omega-6 and 8 per cent omega-3) and rapeseed oil (20 per cent and 10 per cent respectively).

**Oily marine foods:** while land species of plants and animals are predominantly rich in omega-6 fatty acids, marine life forms are higher in omega-3 fatty acids.

**Green vegetables:** although vegetables are not high in fat, the fat they contain is relatively high in omega-3 fatty acids, providing much of the omega-3 in our diet.

# Hydrogenated fats

The high proportion of polyunsaturated fatty acids in a fat has two important consequences: it makes the fat liquid at room temperature (i.e. an oil), and it makes the fat more unstable and liable to become rancid.

When vegetable and fish oils are hardened (hydrogenated) to make margarines and solid cooking fats, some of the unsaturated fats are converted into saturated fats. Some of the remaining unsaturated fat also changes its chemical structure into a 'trans' rather than the natural 'cis' form of fatty acid.

These trans fatty acids have become the focus of attention recently because of the increase in amount in the average diet of people in industrialised countries. It is thought that the body uses them in the same way as saturated fat, and the Department of Health, in their report on diet and prevention of heart disease (1984), recommended that trans fatty acids should be regarded as equivalent to saturated fats for the purpose of dietary recommendations. Although that report recommended that manufacturers should label their products, stating trans fat content as well as total fat, saturated and polyunsaturated fats, it now seems unlikely that the Ministry of Agriculture Fisheries and Food will insist on this because, they say, there is insufficient evidence of adverse effects on health. Trans fats also occur naturally in the fat and milk of multi-stomached animals that chew the cud, including cattle and sheep.

# Average daily intakes

According to a government survey of almost 2,200 British adults (1990), the average intake of fat for men was 102g per day and for women, 74g per day. This accounted for about 40 per cent of the both the men's and women's energy intake from food.

102g fat = 4.4oz margarine OR
3.5ml oil OR
14oz pork pie (three individual pork pies) OR
average spread of butter on seven toasted crumpets.

The Committee on Medical Aspects of Food Policy on Dietary Reference Values (1991) recommended that individuals' total fat intake should not exceed 35 per cent of their food energy from fat, but only 12 per cent of men and 15 per cent of women fell within these recommendations. This means that most of us are eating too much fat.

## Sources of fat in the UK diet

Some fats are obvious, such as butter, margarine, oil, lard and the fat on meat. Less obvious sources include fat in milk, cheese, cream, eggs, fish, nuts, seeds and foods made with fat, such as biscuits, cakes, pastries, crisps and chocolate. Fruit and vegetables are generally low in fat, with the exceptions of avocado pears and olives. The chart below shows the main sources of fat in the UK diet.

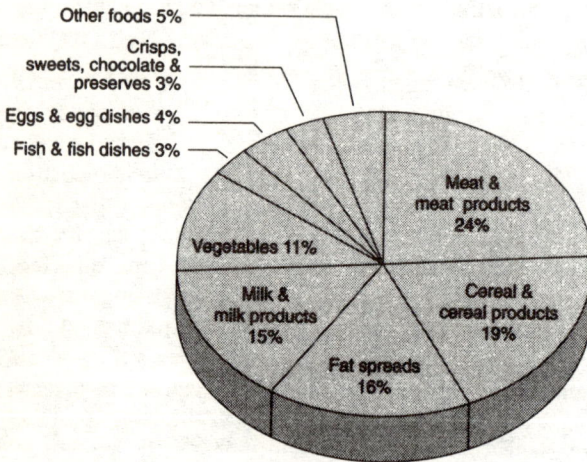

Sources of fat in the UK diet (British Adult Survey, 1990)

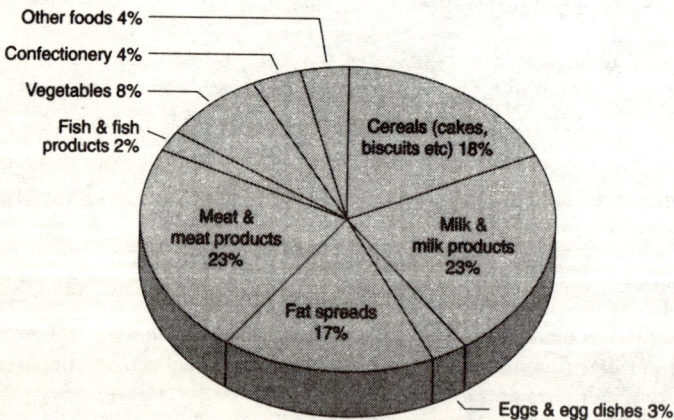

Sources of saturated fat in the UK diet (British Adult Survey, 1990)

## *Fat substitutes*

Fat gives foods such as ice-cream and mayonnaise their creamy taste and texture. Food technologists have now developed substitutes for fat which mimic the 'mouth-feel' and taste, but contain few or no calories. Fat substitutes fall into two categories: calorie-reduced fat substitutes, such as Simplesse, and chemically altered fats that cannot be digested, such as Olestra.

Calorie-reduced or imitation fats are usually made from normal foods such as egg white and milk protein. They are mechanically blended protein particles and usually contain less than 2 calories per gram. Products like Simplesse are only available for use by food manufacturers. Because they cannot be heated, they can only be used in making products such as mayonnaise, ice-cream and margarines.

Chemically altered fats have no nutritional value since they cannot be absorbed. These products can be heated and can be used for many more foods than Simplesse. It is intended that these products, such as Olestra, be used as a fat substitute in foods such as cake mixes, biscuits, chocolate and as a substitute for cooking oil. These chemically altered fats are classified as food additives and have not yet been approved for food use by the government. Concern has been voiced by nutritionists because chemically altered fats interfere with absorption of fat-soluble vitamins.

# Protein

The word 'protein' was coined in 1838 by a Dutch chemist called Mulder, who derived the name from a Greek word meaning 'of first importance'. It is the fundamental structural element of every cell in the body and, historically, it was the first substance recognised as being essential to all living tissues.

Like fat and carbohydrate, protein contains carbon, hydrogen and oxygen, but in addition, it also contains nitrogen and sulphur. Nitrogen is the element that distinguishes tissue-building protein from the other two macronutrients, fat and carbohydrate. If, as most of us do in Western society, you eat more protein than your body needs, the excess nitrogen is excreted in your urine as urea, and the rest of the protein molecule is used for energy or converted to fat and stored, as fat, in the body. The kidneys of most healthy individuals can cope with an excess of nitrogen without difficulty but for those who have kidney damage, the job of excreting unneeded nitrogen can overburden the kidneys, and this is why people with kidney disease are sometimes put on a low protein diet.

Many millions of people in Third World countries are deficient in protein and suffer from a disease called 'kwashiorkor'. Their appearance is deceptive because, although malnourished, they have pot bellies, swollen limbs and puffy faces due to abnormal fluid retention. Because protein is essential for the immune system, kwashiorkor sufferers are very susceptible to infections of all kinds.

## Amino acids

Just as the structural units of fats are fatty acids, the structural units of protein are amino acids. Again, like fatty acids, it is convenient to divide these into two types: essential and non-essential. Essential amino acids cannot be made in the body in sufficient quantities to meet requirements, and have to be obtained from food. There are about 20 common amino acids, of which nine are essential:

| | |
|---|---|
| Isoleucine | Phenylalinine |
| Leucine | Threonine |
| Lysine | Tryptophan |
| Methionine | Valine |
| Histidine | |

Histidine is essential for the rapidly growing infant and has only recently been shown to be required by adults, too.

## Protein functions

Protein is quantitatively more important than either carbohydrate and fat, in that one can live with very small amounts of carbohydrate without any observable ill effects, and although fat is not quite so indispensable, one can live for some time without it. However, there is a minimum protein quantity that is required in order to remain healthy.

Protein plays both structural and functional roles. In its structural role, it is essential in the formation of muscle, bones, skin and hair. Functionally, it is needed for a number of roles including hormone formation, enzyme action and in defence mechanisms. For example, insulin, the hormone that controls blood sugar, is a protein. This is why some diabetics need to have insulin injections rather than take it in pill form. If it were taken orally, it would, as a protein, be broken down and digested as any other protein and would not then be able to regulate blood sugar. Antibodies that defend against disease are proteins. Blood clotting is dependent on protein, as is the transport of oxygen and carbon dioxide around the body. In their role as enzymes, proteins control the breakdown of food for energy, and maintenance and repair of body tissues. When protein is supplied in amounts greater than necessary for growth, maintenance and repair, it will contribute to the energy pool of the body. Similarly, if carbohydrates and fats are not sufficient to meet energy demands, protein will be diverted for that purpose.

## Nutritional value of protein

The nutritional value of a protein food is judged by its ability to provide both the quality and quantity of essential amino acids that the body needs. In general, protein from animal sources – meat, fish, eggs, milk and cheese – is a good source of essential amino acids. Vegetable and cereal sources of protein include pulses (lentils, soyabeans, chickpeas, kidney beans, and other dried beans and peas), bread and other wheat products, nuts and seeds. These sources of protein tend to be low in one or more of the essential amino acids. Wheat, for example, is low in lysine, while beans are low in methionine. It is therefore important that vegetarians, and in particular vegans, eat a variety of different types of plant protein foods. Combinations such as rice and nuts, bread with nuts, hummous with chickpeas and sesame seeds ensure a supply of all the essential amino acids.

## Protein requirements

The Reference Nutrient Intakes for protein, as recommended by the Department of Health (1991), for men and women aged between 19 and 50 is 55.5g and 45g per day respectively. This represents approximately 9 per cent of their energy.

55.5g protein = 3 pints milk OR
8oz cheese OR
7oz lean roast beef

For infants and children, proportionately more is allowed in relation to their size to satisfy growth requirements, and for pregnant and breast-feeding women, additional allowances are made for foetal development and to allow adequate breast milk production. These recommendations are made on the assumption that energy requirements are being met by fat and carbohydrate so that the protein can be used more specifically for growth, maintenance and repair of body tissues.

Animal protein foods have traditionally been synonymous with affluence. Approximately two-thirds of our protein comes from animals, especially meat, an expensive and prestigious food. These high protein foods – meat, cheese and milk – tend to be high in the type of fat most experts say we eat too much of, i.e. saturated fat. To help reduce the amount of saturated fat, there is now a consensus among nutritionists that we should eat less animal protein and more protein from plant foods such as beans, cereal foods like bread and pasta, potatoes, seeds and nuts. Animal protein does, however, contain some very valuable vitamins, especially B vitamins and trace elements such as easily absorbed iron and zinc. A good compromise is, therefore, to choose leaner cuts of meat and reduced/low fat alternatives for milk and cheese. Fish is the healthiest high protein food because:

- white fish contains very little fat and
- those fish that do contain fat (oily fish such as mackerel) contain mostly the health-promoting polyunsaturated fats.

**Average daily intakes**

According to a government survey of almost 2,200 British adults (1990), the average intake of protein for men was 85g per day and for women, 62g per day. This accounted for 15 per cent of the men's energy intake from food and 16 per cent of women's intake.

## Sources of protein in the UK diet

About two-thirds of our protein comes from animal sources and one-third from vegetable and sources.

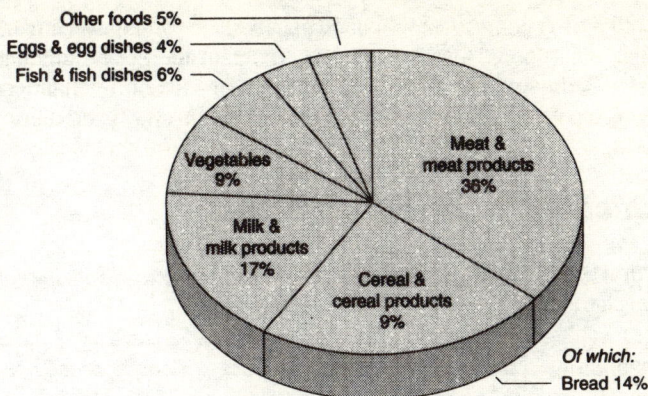

Other foods 5%
Eggs & egg dishes 4%
Fish & fish dishes 6%
Vegetables 9%
Milk & milk products 17%
Cereal & cereal products 9%
Meat & meat products 36%
Of which: Bread 14%

Sources of protein in the UK diet (British Adult Survey, 1990)

# Carbohydrate

Carbohydrate is a term used to cover a whole range of substances, from simple carbohydrates or sugars through to complex carbohydrates which consist of starches and non-starch polysaccharides (fibre). Like fats, they are made up of carbon, hydrogen and oxygen but differ from fats in that hydrogen and oxygen are in the same proportion as found in water, hence the term carbohydrate. Their major function is to provide energy to various tissues, especially to the brain and nervous system which cannot make use of other nutrients for energy purposes. Carbohydrates provide the majority of calories in most cultures, varying from as much as 90 per cent in the diets of poor people, such as in the tropics, to around 40 per cent in more affluent countries such as the UK.

With the exception of the sugar found in milk (lactose), most of the carbohydrate in our diet originates from plant sources. In nature, most carbohydrates occur 'packaged' in foods, for example in grains such as oats or barley, vegetables such as carrots or peas, and fruit such as bananas. In their natural state, these carbohydrates are relatively rich in vitamins and minerals in relation to their calorie content. They are also rich sources of non-starch polysaccharides or fibre. At the turn of the century, most of the carbohydrate in our diet would have been nutrient-rich complex carbohydrates, as in grains and pulses, and natural simple carbohydrates from fruits and vegetables. Today, a high proportion of our carbohydrates comes from foods high in refined, processed sugars. These high-sugar foods, many of which also contain appreciable amounts of fat, are relatively low in essential nutrients in relation to their high calorie content. Hence they are often referred to as 'empty' calories.

## Classification of carbohydrates

Carbohydrates are usually classified as monosaccharides, disaccharides or polysaccharides:

| Carbohydrate | Type | End product of digestion | Food sources |
|---|---|---|---|
| Monosaccharides | glucose<br>fructose<br>galactose | glucose<br>fructose<br>galactose | fruit and honey<br>fruit and honey<br>constituent of lactose |
| Disaccharides | sucrose<br><br>lactose<br><br>maltose | glucose and fructose<br>glucose and galactose<br>glucose and glucose | table sugar<br><br>milk and milk products<br>malt products and some breakfast cereals |
| Polysaccharides (digestible) | starch and dextrins | glucose | grains, tubers and pulses |
| Polysaccharides (non-starch) | cellulose<br>hemicellulose<br>pectin<br>gums<br><br>lignin | not absorbed<br>not absorbed<br>not absorbed<br>not absorbed<br><br>not absorbed | (stalks and leaves of veg; outer seed cover fruits)<br>plant secretions and seeds<br>plant cell walls |

## Sugars

### Monosaccharides

The simplest forms of carbohydrate with which we are concerned in human nutrition are the simple or single sugars (the monosaccharides) glucose, fructose and galactose. Glucose occurs naturally in fruits (notably grapes), honey, sweetcorn and some root vegetables. Most carbohydrates are ultimately broken down to glucose when digested. It is, therefore, the best form of sugar when an immediate supply of energy is needed in disease or for energy purposes. Fructose is found, together with glucose, in honey and fruit. Galactose does not occur free in nature but is a component of lactose (milk sugar).

## Disaccharides

Disaccharides are made up of two monosaccharides linked together, the most important of which are sucrose, lactose and maltose. Sucrose is ordinary table sugar, processed from sugar cane and sugar beet. It also occurs to a lesser extent in fruit and in vegetables such as carrots. Lactose occurs only in milk and milk products such as yoghurt. Although uncommon, some babies have a deficiency of the enzyme lactase, which is necessary to digest lactose, and are said to be 'lactose intolerant'. Maltose is formed when starch is broken down by digestion and in the production of malted beers from grains such as barley.

## Sugar in manufactured foods

Sweetness of taste has given sugars their prominence in human nutrition. The degree of sweetness varies depending on the sugar content, the intensity decreasing in the order of fructose, sucrose, glucose, maltose and galactose and lactose. Brown and white sugars are only part of a whole spectrum of sugars used as sweetening agents. Sweeteners likely to appear on food and drink labels include:

Sucrose, invert sugar, raw cane sugar
Glucose, glucose syrup, dextrose, corn syrup
Syrup, honey, treacle, molasses
Fructose, maltose.

Sugars in fruit and honey have always been a part of man's diet, but sugar only became a substantial part of the UK diet in the middle of the last century when sugar extracted from sugar cane (sucrose) became cheap and available in an easily transportable form. Sucrose (table sugar) now accounts for about one-seventh of our energy intake. On average, each of us in the UK eats almost 100lb of sugar each year – 30 teaspoons a day! This is hardly surprising when you find that there are four teaspoons in a carton of fruit yoghurt, seven teaspoons in a can of Coke, two to three teaspoons in a small tin of baked beans, about five teaspoons in a small tin of fruit in syrup, 20 teaspoons in 4oz boiled sweets and almost ten teaspoons in a regular size chocolate bar. It is also present in many brands of breakfast cereals, sauces, pickles, tinned meats, soups, tinned vegetables such as peas and kidney beans, tinned ravioli, peanut butter and salads such as coleslaw. There are also, of course, the more obvious sources such as cakes, biscuits, ice-cream, chocolate, sweets, puddings, sweetened fizzy drinks, squashes, jams and marmalades. Try to spare the time to compare the list of ingredients on tinned or packet foods you normally buy. Remember, however, that ingredients are listed in order of amount in a product and some products may be sweetened with more than one sugar, allowing each to be listed perhaps lower down the list than would happen if only one source of sugar was used.

## Sugar – brown or white?

There is no particular nutritional merit in brown sugar over white. Apart from calories, neither have nutrients of any significance and they both contain the same amount of calories – a 5g teaspoon contains approximately 19 calories – empty calories containing no vitamins, minerals, fibre, protein or starch.

## Honey

Although honey has acquired a special reputation as a nutritious food, this reputation is overstated. It does contain small amounts of minerals including potassium, calcium and phosphorus, but these are present in such small amounts that they have little significance to human nutrition.

## New terminology for sugars

Experts believe that, from a physiological viewpoint, it is helpful to make a distinction between sugars that are naturally integrated into the cellular structure of a food ('intrinsic') and those which are free in the food or added to it ('extrinsic'). This difference in physical location influences their availability for bacterial breakdown in the mouth and the readiness with which they are absorbed after ingestion.

Although lactose, which occurs naturally in milk, is an extrinsic sugar, it does not contribute to dental caries and therefore should be considered separately from other extrinsic sugars. This has led to a new term – 'non-milk extrinsic sugars' (NMEs) – which will replace the more familiar terms of 'added sugars' or 'refined sugars'. NMEs are principally sucrose and are dubbed by some as 'enemies' because of their association with dental problems.

## Sugar and health

With the widespread use of sugar in our diet have come claims that it is responsible for many of our common ailments. It has been linked with an increased prevalence of dental caries, obesity, diabetes, heart disease and behavioural problems. Most of these claims have been contested, and in some cases, it is difficult to distinguish between fact and vested interests. However, the Department of Health, in its expert committee report on dietary sugars and disease (1989), concluded that, apart from lactose in milk, extrinsic sugars (principally sucrose) do contribute to the development of dental caries. This related not just to the amount consumed but also the frequency with which it was consumed. They also concluded that dietary sugars may contribute to an excess of calorie consumption responsible for obesity, and although sugar played no direct causal role in the development of heart disease, high blood pressure or diabetes, obesity itself played a role in these diseases. They did not believe that sugar had a significant effect on behaviour. In general terms, concern was voiced that there was a trend towards lower vitamin and mineral intakes in those whose diets contained a high sugar content, particularly if their overall calorie intake was low.

# Polysaccharides – complex carbohydrates

Complex carbohydrates consist of polysaccharides (starches) and non-starch polysaccharides (NSP). The latter term, although not entirely interchangeable, replaces the more familiar term, dietary 'fibre'.

## Starches

Starchy foods, such as potatoes, bread, rice, pasta, green bananas, cornmeal, cassava and plantains, form the staple food in most countries. They are an important part of our diet because they are filling without containing too many calories, and because they are generally cheap to buy. Starches are encased within the plant cells by cellulose walls in the form of granules. In this form they are insoluble in water and not usually eaten raw. When cooked in the presence of water, foods such as potatoes and grains become more easily digested. The average daily intake of starch in the UK for men is around 156g compared to 106g per day for women.

In the past, it has been generally believed that starchy foods are fattening. This is not true if they are eaten as they occur in nature, but they can absorb substantial amounts of fat in cooking as, for instance, in chips: a 100g (3.5oz) boiled potato contains about 80 kilocalories, while the same weight of chips will contain over three times that amount – 250 kilocalories.

## Non-starch polysaccharides – fibre

Scientists now favour the term non-starch polysaccharides (NSP) in favour of 'dietary fibre'. This is because it is a more precise chemical definition for most of the compounds which have, in the past, been known as fibre.

Non-starch polysaccharides are structural components of the cell walls of all plants and include cellulose, hemicellulose, pectin, lignin and gums, each of which has its own chemical and physical properties. They are found in all plant foods including cereals and vegetables, especially pulses, fruits, nuts and seeds. In general, NSP are not digested by the human body and so do not contribute significantly to energy intake.

Fibre is sometimes divided into two categories – soluble and insoluble. Soluble fibre is found in oats, pulses, fruit such as apples (pectin) and leafy vegetables. It is thought to be important in helping to reduce blood cholesterol levels and in some forms of diabetes because it slows down absorption of sugars in the blood. Insoluble fibre is the type found in cereal products and has more of a laxative effect.

Appendix 4 gives the NSP content of a number of different foods. In Britain, 50 per cent of NSP is provided by vegetables and 40 per cent by cereals. The average intake of NSP in the UK is approximately 12.5g per day.

12.5g NSP = 17 slices thick-cut white bread OR
4 slices thick-cut wholemeal bread OR
6 Shredded Wheat or Weetabix

The average intake for the adult population should be 18g per day (individual range 12 to 24g per day).

Foods rich in NSP tend to be more bulky and less calorie-dense than foods low in or free of NSP and they require longer to chew. Because high NSP foods are generally high in vitamins and minerals (wholegrain cereals, vegetables and fruit), a diet high in NSP is often indicative of a nutrient-dense diet. Diets low in NSP tend to be high in fat and sugar. For all of these reasons, many popular and successful slimming diets such as the F-Plan Diet are based on this principle.

## NSP and health

There was at one time concern that a high fibre intake reduced the absorption of minerals such as calcium, iron and zinc. This occurs because they bind with fibre-associated substances such as phytate. However, it is generally agreed now that the differences seem too small to pose a serious mineral deficiency, and any reduction in vitamin absorption is likely to be compensated by the higher levels of vitamins generally contained in high fibre foods.

Diets low in NSP have been associated with an increased risk of constipation, diverticulitis, bowel cancer, obesity, heart disease, diabetes and gallstones. However, experts believe that the protective effect of NSP *per se* is inconclusive. Even where the evidence is strongest, it has not been possible to adequately separate the effects of NSP from those of other components of the diet such as calories, fat, vitamins and minerals. A further problem is that NSP is used to define a complex mixture of substances, and analysis of studies in terms of total NSP content could be misleading if the effect of one component masks the effect of another. However, consistent results have shown that a diet high in NSP (especially fruit and vegetables) and relatively low in fat is beneficial in some diseases. Although it is not known whether this is due to the high NSP content of the diet or to variations in other dietary components, such as vitamins, it is thought reasonable to recommend an increase in our current dietary levels of NSP.

## Average daily intakes

According to a government survey of British adults (1990), the average intake of carbohydrate for men was 272g per day and for women, 193g per day. This accounted for around 45 per cent of their respective energy intakes from food.

272g carbohydrate = 10 thick-cut slices bread (544g) OR
4 large jacket potatoes (850g)

## *Sources of carbohydrate*

In the 1990 survey of British adults, almost half (46 per cent) of the total carbohydrate came from cereal products, with bread contributing 22 per cent of total intake.

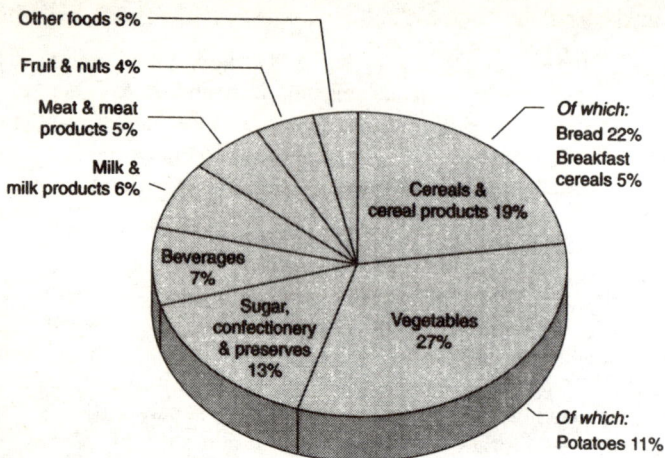

Other foods 3%
Fruit & nuts 4%
Meat & meat products 5%
Milk & milk products 6%
Beverages 7%
Sugar, confectionery & preserves 13%
Vegetables 27%
Cereals & cereal products 19%
Of which: Bread 22% Breakfast cereals 5%
Of which: Potatoes 11%

Sources of carbohydrate in the UK diet (British Adult Survey, 1990)

## A summary of advice on carbohydrates

### Cut down on sugars

- Stop adding sugar to tea and coffee.
- Cut down on biscuits, cakes, sweets and chocolates.
- Choose unsweetened/low sugar varieties of fizzy drinks and fruit juice.
- Have fresh fruit instead of puddings.
- Choose breakfast cereals with a low sugar content.
- Compare ingredient lists and nutrition information on different brands of similar products.

### Increase starches

- Eat at least four to six slices of bread a day.
- Eat more cereal foods of all kinds.
- Replace sugary and fatty foods with more bread, potatoes, pasta and rice.
- Bulk up stews with root vegetables and pulses such as kidney beans.

### Increase non-starch polysaccharides

- Choose the wholegrain varieties of bread, rice and pasta.

- Compare the nutrition labels on breakfast cereals and choose those with a high NSP/fibre content.
- Eat more vegetables and fruit.

## Alcohol

For many people, drinking alcohol is a pleasant social pastime and, as long as it is kept within sensible limits, it is unlikely to cause any harm. However, it is important to be aware of its possible detrimental effects. It is high in calories, providing 7 kilocalories per gram of neat alcohol. This is less than the 9 kilocalories found in every gram of fat but considerably more than the 3.75 and 4 kilocalories found respectively in carbohydrate and protein.

Alcohol has to be considered a nutrient because it supplies usable energy. It has, however, been called the anti-nutrient nutrient: distilled spirits contain nothing but energy – no vitamins, minerals or any other nutrient. Beer, stout and wine do contain some vitamins and minerals, as well as carbohydrate, but the amounts are too small to be of any nutritional significance. To compound the issue, alcohol interferes with the absorption of some vitamins, in particular folic acid and vitamin B12. It also deprives the body of nutrients from other foods, because the liver requires vitamins to break alcohol down to energy, which means these vitamins have to come from other sources and are not available for other essential purposes. Since alcohol has a diuretic effect, i.e. it increases the output of urine, it can cause a loss in water-soluble minerals such as zinc, potassium and magnesium.

What this means is that not only does alcohol not contribute any essential nutrients to the diet, it also increases one's requirements for many nutrients. This may not be a problem for a light or even moderate imbiber, providing they are getting sufficient essential nutrients from other sources and that alcohol is not causing a weight problem from excess calories. However, people who drink heavily tend not to eat regularly or eat well. The toxic effects of alcohol are then compounded by malnutrition, aggravated by increased nutrient requirements and perhaps, in extreme circumstances, a decreased ability of the liver to metabolise any nutrients.

## Alcohol content

The alcohol and calorie content of alcoholic beverages is given below, per pub measure.

|  | Amount | Alcohol | Kcals |
|---|---|---|---|
| **Spirits** (40% by volume) | ¼ gill (1 English pub measure) | 7.6 | 53 |
| **Beers** |  |  |  |
| Lager | ½ pint | 9.0 | 82 |
| Bitter | ½ pint | 8.8 | 90 |
| Stout | ½ pint | 8.2 | 105 |
| **Cider** |  |  |  |
| Dry | ½ pint | 10.7 | 102 |
| **Wines** | 1 glass |  |  |
| Red | (125ml) | 11.9 | 85 |
| White, dry | (125ml) | 11.4 | 83 |
| White, sweet | (125ml) | 12.7 | 117 |
| Champagne | (125ml) | 12.4 | 95 |
| **Fortified wines** | small glass |  |  |
| Sherry, dry | (50ml) | 7.8 | 58 |
| Sherry, sweet | (50ml) | 7.8 | 68 |
| Port | (50ml) | 8.0 | 79 |

Data/information from *The Composition of Foods*, 5th ed. (1991) is reproduced with the permission of the Royal Society of Chemistry and the Controller of HMSO.

## Recommended maximum intake

The generally agreed safe upper limit per week is 21 units for men and 14 units for women, with one or two alcohol-free days per week. One unit of alcohol, as defined by the Health Education Authority, is approximately 10g alcohol and equates to approximately half a pint of ordinary beer, one glass of wine or one pub measure of spirits such as whisky, gin, vodka or brandy. It should be remembered when 'totting up' units that measures served at home tend to be considerably more generous than pub measures and, if purchased outside the UK, may contain more than 40 per cent alcohol by volume (see label).

The current advice to pregnant women and women anticipating pregnancy is to cut out alcohol, especially around the time you plan to conceive and during the first three months of pregnancy, or at least try to limit it to four units per week. If you are breast feeding, remember alcohol can be passed on to your baby through your breast milk.

Excessive alcohol consumption increases the risk of high blood pressure, cirrhosis of the liver, alcoholic brain damage as well as various cancers. Balanced against this there is some evidence that low levels of alcohol (10–20g alcohol a day) may have beneficial effects, including some reduction in the risk of coronary heart disease and of cholesterol gallstone formation.

## Intake

The Survey of British Adults (1990) reported that 79 per cent of men and 65 per cent of women drank alcohol during the week they recorded their intakes. The average daily intake of male consumers was 31.5g. This represents around 21 units a week which is an acceptable level for men. However, since some men do not drink at all and some drink only very occasionally, it does mean some were drinking more than may be good for their health. Women consumers had about a third of the average intake of men (10.6g/day). This represented 8.7 per cent and 4.3 per cent of their total kilocalorie intake respectively.

### Tips on how to keep within the limit

- Allow yourself 14 units of alcohol each week if you are a woman, 21 if a man and have one or two alcohol-free days each week.
- If you drink wine with meals, have two glasses – one for water.
- Extend alcoholic drinks by adding mineral water or other mixers to your wine or other drinks.
- Drink more slowly; drinking round for round can make you increase the pace at which you drink – avoid getting involved in buying rounds.
- Alternate low alcohol drinks with alcoholic drinks.
- Make your drinks smaller – buy a spirit measure for home use. Order halves instead of pints.
- Try to disassociate drinking alcohol from certain occasions which have become habit.

# 2
# VITAMINS AND MINERALS

## ——— Vitamins ———

Vitamins are a collection of potent organic substances which help to regulate the chemical processes that occur in the body and are essential to life. Most vitamins cannot be made in the body and so have to be obtained from food or food supplements. Vitamins are distinguishable from minerals by virtue of their organic nature. They are required in only minute amounts: human requirements for each vitamin range from 1mcg to 1mg per day (see Appendix 7).

Each vitamin plays its own unique part, and each is important for specific functions such as vision, blood clotting, health of the skin or the skeleton. They also have a general function in helping to regulate the breakdown of protein, fat and/or carbohydrate into energy and to assist in the absorption of minerals from food.

Vitamins are classified into two groups: fat soluble (A, D, E and K) and water soluble (eight B vitamins and vitamin C). Water-soluble vitamins are required daily because the body has a limited ability to store most of them. Water-soluble vitamins are normally excreted in the urine if more is consumed than required by the body. Fat-soluble vitamins can be stored in the body, especially by the liver. For this reason, it is less important to have a source of these every day. Mineral oils, such as liquid paraffin, interfere with the absorption of fat-soluble vitamins. For this reason, long-term use of such a laxative is not recommended.

# *Do we need supplements? What the experts say . . .*

Millions of pounds are spent in the UK every year on multivitamin and mineral supplements by the public, who continue to believe unerringly in their beneficial effects. There has, for example, been a persistently held belief that vitamin C will help prevent colds, but an analysis of 27 controlled studies showed that vitamin C has no worthwhile effect in preventing colds. In the nutrition survey of British adults, 17 per cent of women and 9 per cent of men were taking a food supplement.

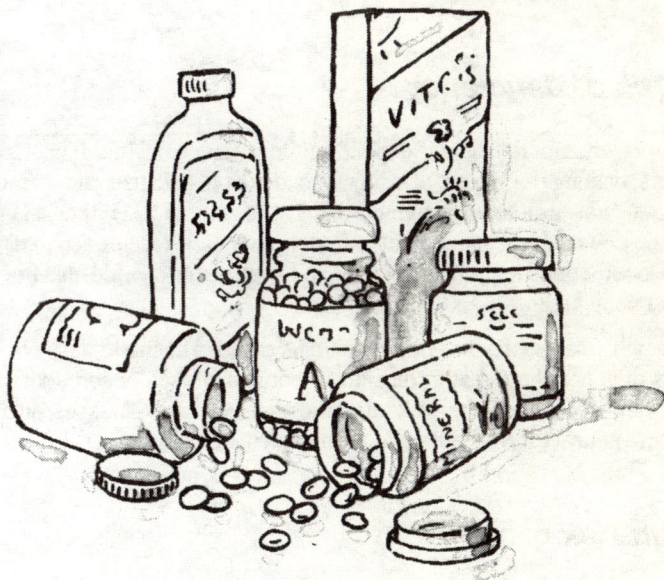

Expert committees are sceptical about the benefits of vitamin/mineral supplements, at least in relation to those living in affluent societies. The USA National Research Council reported that it could find no evidence that daily vitamin/mineral supplements (equalling no more than the Recommended Daily Allowances) were either beneficial or harmful for the general population. A letter in the *British Medical Journal* stated, 'the consensus is clear: healthy adult men and healthy non-pregnant women consuming a normal varied diet do not need vitamin supplements'. This, of course, begs the question, what is 'a normal healthy diet'?

### Interdependence of micronutrients

The activities of many vitamins and minerals are interrelated and they function most efficiently when ingested in the correct proportions. For example, some nutrients compete for absorption, and if a large dose is taken of one, it can reduce the absorption of another, as for example happens with calcium and zinc. Similarly, some nutrients enhance the absorption of others, as in the cases of vitamin C and iron or vitamin D and calcium. Therefore, taking supplements of one without the other may be ineffectual or even harmful. The expert committee who recommended the daily reference values will have taken these interrelationships into account and so indicated the proportions in which they should be provided. See Appendix 7.

## Signs of deficiency

Signs of vitamin deficiency depend on how 'deficiency' is defined. If it means waiting for signs of scurvy to develop because of vitamin C deficiency or beri-beri through low intakes of thiamin (B1), then it is true that obvious clinical signs of vitamin deficiency are rare in economically developed countries which account for approximately one-third of the world population.

However, marginal deficiency in vitamins can lead to subtle, less obvious signs of ill health, and at a third level, optimal intakes of some vitamins may help to reduce the risk of some diseases and illnesses such as cancer, neural tube defects and premenstrual tension.

## High-risk groups

Even when there is an adequate or even surplus supply of food, inappropriate eating patterns or food choices can lead to vitamin deficiencies. Those most likely to be deficient in vitamins include the following.

- Low-income groups, where inappropriate food choices are likely to have a greater impact than on those who are more affluent;
- The elderly, who may not be consuming enough food in general, perhaps because of poor appetite or because food choices are restricted to easily prepared foods like tea and biscuits. Those who are housebound and not benefiting from exposure to sunlight may have low vitamin D levels.

- Pregnant and breast-feeding women, where there is an increased requirement for many nutrients.
- Chronic 'slimmers' and anorexics (who suffer from an obsessional fear of fatness), who restrict their energy and consequently their micronutrient intakes.
- Alcoholics, whose eating patterns are often poor, whose requirements for some nutrients will be increased to cope with alcohol consumption and whose ability to utilise nutrients is diminished because of liver and other organ malfunctions.
- The chronically sick, either because of gut malabsorption, lack of appetite or increased requirements.
- Vegans, who run a risk of being deficient in vitamin B12. They should, therefore, eat enriched products such as fortified breakfast cereals, meat substitutes, soya milk and yeast extracts.
- People with a suppressed immune system, either drug-induced or because of various infections, most notably the AIDS virus. Some cancers, such as leukaemia, also suppress the immune system.

## Preserving vitamins in food

Vitamins are sensitive to environmental conditions such as heat, light, water and air. They are affected by food storage time, processing and cooking. The most vulnerable vitamins are vitamin C, folic acid and thiamin (B1), but losses also occur with riboflavin (B2), pyridoxine (B6), vitamin B12, vitamin A and vitamin E. Losses can be reduced by correct storage and cooking.

### Tips on how to preserve vitamins in food

- Never soak vegetables and fruit. Remember, many vitamins are soluble in water and will leach out if food is left in water, especially if chopped.
- Cook vegetables for as short a time as possible and in very little water. Much better to microwave, steam or stir-fry them.
- Add vegetables to water that is already boiling to cut down cooking time.
- Serve cooked vegetables as soon as possible.
- Buy fresh vegetables and fruit when you plan to eat them. The longer the time between picking and eating, the lower the vitamin content. Frozen food is often higher in nutrients than fresh food kept for more

than a few days or kept under inappropriate conditions (see pages 79–80).
- Do not thaw frozen vegetables before cooking. Frozen vegetables retain more nutrients than tinned.
- Eat raw vegetables and fruit where possible.

## Vitamin A (Retinol and Carotene)

### Functions
Vitamin A is essential for a healthy skin, mucous membranes and healthy eyes, protecting against poor vision in dim light (night blindness) and general eye disorders. It is also involved in immune responses to infection.

A high intake of carotene is thought to provide some protection against cancer. High intakes of fruit and vegetables have been associated with a low incidence of some forms of cancer but, as yet, it has not been proved that carotene is the protective factor.

### Sources
Vitamin A is found in animal foods as retinol and plant foods as beta-carotene, called a precursor of vitamin A. The richest natural sources of retinol are fish liver oils such as cod liver oil. It is also very concentrated in animal livers. Because of changes in animal feeding practices, the vitamin A content has more than doubled in lamb's, pig's and calf's liver in the past 20 years. It has increased substantially in ox and chicken liver (see section on excessive intakes). Retinol is also found in some fatty fish, such as mackerel and herring, egg yolk, full fat milk, butter, cheese and fortified margarine.

Vitamin A can be made in the body from carotene. Carotene is found in fruit and vegetables, particularly those that are yellow such as carrots and apricots, and dark green vegetables such as spinach and spring greens. However, it is necessary to eat six times as much carotene as retinol to produce the same quantity of vitamin A (6mcg beta-carotene = 1mcg retinol).

### Deficiency
Vitamin A deficiency is rare in developed countries because it can be stored in the liver, and most people will have sufficient to meet their normal requirements for many months without eating more. However, vitamin A deficiency is a common cause of blindness in Third World countries.

## Requirement
Reference Nutrient Intakes (RNI; see page 95) for vitamin A range from 350mcg per day for babies, up to 950mcg for breast-feeding mothers. The normal RNI for adult men and women is 700mcg and 600mcg per day respectively. The average daily intake of the adult UK population is about 1,680mcg for men and 1,490mcg for women.

## Achieving the Reference Nutrient Intake
According to a recent Ministry of Agriculture analysis, there is 38,690mcg of vitamin A in 100g of lamb's liver. This means that a medium-sized portion (100g/3.5oz) of lamb's liver provides enough retinol to satisfy an average woman's needs for vitamin A for 90 weeks. If you prefer not to eat liver, or have been advised not to (see below), then you could satisfy a day's requirements for vitamin A by having a 3.5oz portion of carrots (1,260mcg) or a large mango (750mcg).

## Excessive Intakes
Regular intakes of retinol should not exceed 6,600mcg in adults and 3,300mcg a day if pregnant or thinking of becoming pregnant. There is thought to be an association between high intakes of vitamin A, particularly around the time of conception, and an increased risk of birth defects. As a precaution, women who are, or might become pregnant, have been advised by the Department of Health not to take vitamin A supplements and not to eat liver, because of the large increases in vitamin A concentrations in liver. Large intakes of retinol can cause liver and bone damage and other abnormalities. Carotene is not toxic, although very high intakes can lead to a yellow appearance.

# The B vitamins

This group of vitamins, while they each have distinct roles, tend to function as a team and are generally found in similar foods.

### Vitamin B1 (Thiamin)

#### Functions
Thiamin has been known as the antineuritic vitamin because it is needed for normal functioning of the brain and nervous system. It controls the release of energy from carbohydrate. Thiamin is essential for normal appetite, and digestion.

#### Deficiency
The clinical condition associated with prolonged low thiamin intake is

beri-beri, the symptoms of which involve the nervous system and the heart.

### Sources
Over a third of our thiamin comes from cereal products, including breakfast cereals and bread. Thiamin is also plentiful in lean pork, liver, wholegrain cereals, pulses, peanuts, yeast, milk and eggs.

### Requirement
Requirements are related to the amount of carbohydrate in the diet. The more starch and sugar we eat, the more thiamin we need. The Reference Nutrient Intake for thiamin ranges from 0.2mg per day in infancy to 1.1mg in teenage boys (age 15 to 18 years) whose growth and hence energy requirements are at their peak. The Reference Nutrient Intake for adults is 0.8mg per day for women and 1.0mg for men. The average daily intake for adult men and women is 2.01mg and 1.61mg respectively.

### Achieving the Reference Nutrient Intake
Most peoples' requirements for thiamin will be met with a bowl of fortified breakfast cereal (0.6mg) and four slices of brown or wholemeal bread (0.4mg), or from a medium portion of lean roast pork (0.8mg) and a serving of frozen peas (0.3mg).

## Vitamin B2 (Riboflavin)

### Functions
Riboflavin is essential for the breakdown of carbohydrate, fat and protein into energy. It is involved in enzyme regulating activities, particularly relating to the thyroid gland.

### Deficiency
Obvious signs are rare but include sores at corners of the mouth. Serious deficiency is thought to result in retarded growth.

### Sources
The most valuable source of riboflavin is milk, which supplies about one-third of the average intake in the UK. Other good sources include egg yolk, liver, kidney and heart, cheese, wholemeal bread and cereals and green vegetables. Riboflavin is sensitive to ultraviolet light, and much of the riboflavin in bottled milk can be destroyed if left on the doorstep all day, especially in sunshine.

### Requirement
The Reference Nutrient Intakes for riboflavin range from 0.4mg per day for infants to 1.6mg per day for women who are breast feeding. The RNI

for adults is 1.1mg per day for women and 1.3mg for men. The average daily intake of adult women in the UK is about 1.8mg and of men, 2.3mg.

### Achieving the Reference Nutrient Intake
You can get 1.3mg of riboflavin from half a pint of milk (0.5mg) with a bowl of fortified breakfast cereal (0.8mg). A medium portion (3.5oz) of liver contains 3mg.

## Vitamin B3 (Niacin)

### Functions
Niacin helps to control the release of energy from protein, fat and carbo-hydrate. It is essential for normal growth and for healthy skin.

### Deficiency
The classical deficiency disease is pellegra, which is characterised by the three Ds – dermatitis, diarrhoea and, in extreme cases, dementia.

### Sources
Niacin occurs either preformed in foods or as tryptophan, an essential amino acid, which can be converted to niacin. It takes 60mg of tryptophan to make 1mg of niacin. Niacin is widely distributed in plant and animal foods but in relatively small amounts. About one-third of the total intake in the UK is derived from meat and meat products. Other good sources of niacin include wholemeal bread and cereals, fortified breakfast cereals, fish, pulses, nuts, yeast and meat extracts.

### Requirement
Related to energy intake, the Reference Nutrient Intakes for niacin range from 3mg per day for infants to 18mg per day for adolescent boys with high energy requirements to meet growth demands. The Reference Nutrient Intake for adults is 13mg per day for women and 17mg for men. The average daily intake of niacin equivalents (i.e. preformed niacin plus tryptophan divided by 60) is about 30mg for women and 41mg for men.

### Achieving the Reference Nutrient Intake
A portion of tinned tuna (16mg) and four slices of brown or wholemeal bread (5mg) will meet the Reference Nutrient Intake.

### Excessive intakes
Very high doses of niacin have been associated with liver damage. Regular amounts above 500mg a day are considered to be undesirable.

## Vitamin B5 (Pantothenic Acid)

Pantothenic acid is necessary for the release of energy from food. It is so widely distributed in food that a deficiency is unlikely in humans. Although a lack of pantothenic acid will cause greying of hair in rats, supplements have not prevented humans from developing grey hair! Average daily intakes in the UK are 4.5mg for women and 6.3mcg for men.

## Vitamin B6 (Pyridoxine)

### Functions
Essential for breaking down protein for use in building new body tissue. Pyridoxine is also involved in the production of antibodies and red blood cells. Some, but not all, women find that premenstrual tension is helped by taking large amounts (100mg a day) of B6 (see PMT, page 146).

### Deficiency disease
Gross signs of deficiency are rare. In the 1950s, however, deficiency occurred in infants fed on milk formulas which had undergone severe heat treatment during their manufacture, causing most of the vitamin B6 to be destroyed.

### Sources
Vitamin B6 occurs widely in food, but the best sources are meat, especially liver and pork, and fish. Other reasonable sources include eggs, wholegrain cereals, fortified breakfast cereals, peanuts, bananas, potatoes and other vegetables.

### Requirement
Related to total protein intake, the Reference Nutrient Intakes range from 0.2mg per day in infants to 1.5mg per day in adolescent boys with rapid growth demands. The Reference Nutrient Intake for adults is 1.2mg per day for women and 1.4mg for men. The average daily intake for women in the UK is 2.8mg and for men is 2.7mg.

### Achieving the Reference Nutrient Intake
You can get 1.4mg of vitamin B6 from a portion of cod (0.85mg) with a medium-size portion of potatoes (0.6mg) or a banana (0.6mg).

### Excessive intakes
Amounts above 100mg a day on a regular basis are considered to be undesirable. Amounts in excess of 200–300mg a day have caused severe nerve damage.

## Vitamin B12 (Cyanocobalomin)

### Functions
In 1948, vitamin B12 was found to be the cure for pernicious anaemia. It

plays an important role in red blood cell formation and in the maintenance of the nervous system and bone marrow. It interacts closely with folic acid, another B vitamin.

## Deficiency

Deficiency characteristically leads to pernicious anaemia, and prolonged deficiency can lead to irreversible nerve damage. Deficiency has been observed in some very strict vegetarians and vegans, who obtain essentially no vitamin B12 from food, since B12 occurs only in animal products.

## Sources

Vitamin B12 is unique among vitamins because it is only found in foods of animal origin. Liver is the richest source, but it also occurs in kidney and other meats, oily fish such as sardines and mackerel, milk, cheese and eggs.

## Requirement

Reference Nutrient Intakes range from 0.3mcg per day for infants to 2mcg per day for breast-feeding mothers. The RNI for adults is 1.5mcg per day for women and men. The average daily intake of vitamin B12 for women is 5.4mcg and for men, 7.3mcg.

## Achieving the Reference Nutrient Intake

A medium portion (3.5oz) of lamb's liver provides 81mcg of B12, the same amount of sardines contains 28mcg or an egg, 1.3mcg.

## Folic Acid

### Functions

Folic acid is essential for the formation of red and white blood cells in bone marrow. It also plays an important part, along with vitamin B12, in rapidly dividing cells, as, for instance, very early in pregnancy. It has been found to have a very substantial protective effect against neural tube defects, such as spina bifida, when taken around the time of conception and early in pregnancy.

### Deficiency

The characteristic sign of deficiency is megaloblastic anaemia, sometimes seen in pregnancy. Other rapidly regenerating tissues, such as the mucosa of the intestine, may also suffer, while in babies and young children, growth may be affected.

### Sources

Folic acid occurs in many foods but is especially rich in liver, kidney and in raw green leafy vegetables. It also occurs in reasonable quantities in wholegrain cereals, eggs, pulses, avocado pears, bananas and orange juice. A diet that is rich in other B vitamins and in vitamin C is usually rich in folic acid, too.

## Requirement
The Reference Nutrient Intake ranges from 50mcg per day for infants to 300mcg for pregnant women. The RNI for adults is 200mcg per day. The average intake of folic acid for women is 213mcg and for men, 311mcg.

## Achieving the Reference Nutrient Intake
You can get 300mcg of folic acid from a bowl of fortified breakfast cereal (100mcg) plus two slices of granary bread (50mcg), a serving of spinach (125mcg) plus a serving of baked beans (40mcg), or an orange (40mcg). A medium portion of lamb's liver contains 200mcg.

## Biotin

Biotin is an essential component in many enzyme systems and is necessary for the release of energy from fat. It is widely distributed in food, and deficiency in humans is unlikely, since it is manufactured by bacteria normally inhabiting the large intestine. Average daily intakes in the UK are around 28mcg for women and 39mcg for men.

## Vitamin C (Ascorbic Acid)

### Functions
Vitamin C has numerous functions, including maintenance of healthy skin, blood vessels, gums and teeth, normal wound healing and formation of antibodies, as well as helping iron absorption. It is an important antioxidant, having the ability to destroy harmful free radical substances (see Glossary). It may also play a role in the prevention of some cancers and in lowering blood cholesterol levels.

### Deficiency
Scurvy, characterised by multiple haemorrhages, is one of the oldest diseases known to mankind. It was endemic in Northern Europe in the Middle Ages during winter, when good sources of vitamin C, such as vegetables and fruit, would have been scarce. English sailors came to be known as 'limeys' when early rations included limes, or more correctly lemons, in a successful effort to prevent scurvy. Less extreme deficiency symptoms include tiredness, bleeding gums, delayed wound healing and lowered resistance to infection.

## Sources

Vitamin C, the only other water-soluble vitamin besides the B group, was given a different name because it was found in different foods. The best sources include fresh fruit and vegetables. Rosehips, blackcurrants, strawberries and citrus fruit, such as oranges and grapefruit, and their juices are especially rich, as are raw peppers, tomatoes and green leafy vegetables. Potatoes, although not a concentrated source, are a useful source because of the amount we usually eat. Since vitamin C is water soluble and easily destroyed by heat, foods eaten raw are higher in vitamin C than their cooked equivalents.

## Requirement

Humans, unlike most animals except monkeys and guinea pigs, are unable to make their own vitamin C and are therefore dependent on food for their vitamin C. The Reference Nutrient Intake ranges from 25mg per day for infants to 70mg for breast-feeding mothers. The RNI for adult men and women is 40mg per day. The average intake in the UK, from food sources, is 62mg for women and 66mg for men.

## Achieving the Reference Nutrient Intake

One orange will provide you with 72mg of vitamin C. Alternatively, a serving of broccoli contains 34mg and brussels sprouts, 40mg.

## Excessive amounts

Regular intakes in excess of 6g a day are considered to be undesirable.

## Vitamin D (Calciferol)

## Functions

Vitamin D is essential for normal growth and development and for the formation of bones and teeth. It has an important role in regulating appropriate levels of calcium and phosphorus in the blood to support healthy bone growth and strength.

## Deficiency

Deficiency in childhood leads to rickets, characterised by deformed bones, typically bow-shaped legs, knock-knees and pigeon-chests. In adults, deficiency causes osteomalacia, with softening of the bones causing deformities and fractures. Osteomalacia is most frequently seen in women of child-bearing age who have become depleted of calcium because of multiple pregnancies and inadequate diet, or little exposure to the sun. In both rickets and osteomalacia, a low blood calcium level may result in a form of painful muscle spasm known as tetany.

## Sources

Vitamin D is produced by the action of sunlight on the skin. In the UK, people exposed to sunshine are capable of making enough vitamin D during the summer months to satisfy their requirements for those months and to build up liver stores to last through the winter. For those who are unable to go in the sun, a supply of vitamin D must be obtained from food sources. There are few dietary sources. Fatty fish, such as herring, mackerel, pilchards, sardines and tuna, are a rich source but not eaten in large enough quantities to be a major contributor to the UK diet. Other sources include eggs and fortified foods such as margarine and some milks.

## Requirement

As long as we get sufficient amounts from sunlight, there is no need for a dietary source of vitamin D. However, those who are housebound or who choose to cover their skin may need a dietary supply. The only groups for whom a dietary supply is recommended are infants and young children, those over 65 years old and pregnant and breast-feeding women. Some Asian children, adolescents and women have a relatively higher risk of low vitamin D status due to a combination of their vegetarian diet, low calcium intake and limited exposure to sunshine. For this reason, the expert panel on dietary reference values recommended Asian women and children should take supplementary vitamin D. The Reference Nutrient Intake ranges from 7mcg per day for young children to 10mcg for the elderly and pregnant and lactating women. The average intake of vitamin D for adults is about 3mcg per day.

## Achieving the Reference Nutrient Intake

One mackerel will provide 46mcg of vitamin D, or a kipper, 31mcg.

## Excessive amounts

Large amounts over a period of time can lead to calcification of soft tissues including kidneys, heart and around joints. This is because vitamin D is responsible for absorption of calcium. Regular amounts above 50mcg a day are undesirable.

## Vitamin E (Tocopherol)

## Functions

Vitamin E has a powerful antioxidant effect, preventing the oxidation or destruction of other essential nutrients such as essential fatty acids and vitamin A. There is some evidence that increased tissue levels of vitamin E may protect against heart disease and cancer, but further research is needed in this area.

### Sources
Vitamin E is present in small quantities in many plants, especially seed oils and the outer germ of cereals. It is also found in seeds, peanuts, green plants, milk and milk products and egg yolks.

### Deficiency
Vitamin E deficiency was seen in premature babies before infant formulae contained adequate vitamin E concentrations. No other group of people has shown signs of deficiency.

### Requirement
Requirements are related to polyunsaturated fatty acid intake. Because this varies widely, it was not thought possible to set Reference Nutrient Intakes of practical value. Instead, a 'safe' intake has been set at more than 4mg for men and 3mg for women. The average daily intake in the UK is about 12mg for men and 9mg for women.

## Vitamin K

### Functions
Known as the anti-haemorrhage vitamin, vitamin K helps to regulate blood clotting.

### Deficiency
Vitamin K deficiency is rarely seen after the first few months of life. Newborn infants are prone to have low reserves of vitamin K and can develop haemorrhagic disease of the newborn, manifesting itself by abnormal bleeding. There is a growing consensus that all newborn babies should be given vitamin K at birth.

### Sources
Vitamin K is found in large amounts in green leafy vegetables, especially broccoli and spinach. It is also found in wheat bran, cheese, egg yolk and liver. In addition, vitamin K is formed by bacterial action in the intestine.

### Requirement
Because vitamin K is made in the intestine, it is not possible to make an accurate estimate of requirements for the normal adult.

# Minerals

Minerals are inorganic substances that perform a wide range of vital functions throughout the body. Depending on the amount present or required in the body, they tend to be referred to as either mineral elements or, in the case of those required in small amounts, trace elements or trace minerals. The minerals required in amounts in excess of about 250mg each day by adults are calcium, phosphorus, magnesium, sodium, chloride and potassium. The trace elements, required in amounts usually less than 15mg each day, include iron, zinc, copper, manganese, iodine, fluoride, chromium, molybdenum, and selenium. There is a long list of other elements found in low concentrations in the body, but there is no evidence that these are essential. They include: aluminium, arsenic, antimony, boron, bromine, cadmium, caesium, cobalt, geranium, lead, lithium, mercury, nickel, silicon, silver, strontium, sulphur, tin and vanadium.

The main functions of minerals are:

● constituents of bones and teeth (for example, calcium, phosphorus and magnesium);
● soluble salts which help control the composition of body fluids (sodium, chloride, potassium, magnesium and phosphorus);
● as essential components of enzymes and other proteins such as haemoglobin (for example, iron and phosphorus).

Although health food shops and chemists' shelves are well stocked with bottles of minerals and trace elements, either individually or as a multi-mineral, they can compete against each other for absorption, particularly if not taken in the proper balance. The best way, therefore, to get your daily supply of minerals and trace elements is from the foods you eat. Apart from possibly iron and zinc, a well-structured and varied diet should provide all that your body requires of these essential nutrients.

Concern has been expressed that a high fibre intake, particularly a high bran intake, will reduce the absorption of minerals such as calcium and zinc. A reduction in absorption can happen when phytic acid, contained in cereals, combines with minerals and prevents them being absorbed. This concern is now thought to be unfounded, because most of the foods that contain phytic acid are also good sources of minerals, thus compensating for any reduction in absorption.

Minerals are more stable and less easily destroyed than vitamins, so little is generally lost in cooking.

## Calcium

Besides ensuring strong and healthy bones, calcium is important as a regulator for normal blood clotting, nerve and muscle function and hormone production. The body needs calcium throughout life, but especially during periods of growth, pregnancy and breast feeding.

## Functions
Calcium is the body's most abundant mineral: 98 per cent of it is present in the bone structure, about 1 per cent in teeth and the remaining 1 per cent is in the soft tissues where it acts as a regulator of important functions including nerve conduction, muscle contraction, blood clotting, control of heart beat, enzyme activation and the secretion of hormones such as insulin. Levels of soft tissue calcium are maintained at the expense of bone when there is inadequate calcium intake or absorption.

Although we tend to think of the skeleton as being fairly inert, it is constantly being renewed. Throughout life, bones go through a continual process of 'remodelling' – replacing old bone for new. An adult's entire skeleton is replaced every seven to ten years; children replace theirs about every two years.

## Deficiency
Loss of calcium from bones is a normal part of ageing, but osteoporosis (porous or brittle bones) occurs when calcium is lost from the bones faster than it is replaced. Women are particularly vulnerable after the menopause or after a hysterectomy because of hormonal changes. However, taking large amounts of calcium in middle age does not prevent bone loss. The best way of avoiding osteoporosis appears to be to have enough calcium to achieve peak bone density by the age of 30. It is, however, important to have an adequate intake throughout life.

## Sources
Milk, cheese and yoghurt are the best sources of calcium. Half a pint of milk (low fat or whole) supplies around 340mg of calcium – half the adult daily requirement. It is difficult to meet the recommended intake without milk and milk products. Other good sources include fish where the bones are eaten, such as tinned sardines and pilchards, dark green leafy vegetables and hard water. Since white flour is fortified with calcium by law, white bread is also a useful source.

## Requirements
The body needs calcium throughout life, but especially during periods of growth, pregnancy and breast feeding. Vitamin D is essential for the absorption of calcium, and when calcium is in short supply, an increase in vitamin D helps to compensate by increasing absorption. The Reference Nutrient Intake (RNI) for calcium varies from 350mg per day for one to three year olds, to 1,250mg for breast-feeding women. 700mg a day are

recommended for adult men and women. The dietary survey of British adults (1990) showed an average calcium intake of 940mg and 730mg per day for men and women respectively.

### Achieving the Reference Nutrient Intake
A daily intake of 700mg can be achieved from half a pint of milk (340mg), 1oz hard cheese (205mg) and four slices of brown or white bread (160mg).

## Phosphorus

### Functions
Phosphorus is the companion nutrient to calcium and comes next to calcium as the second most abundant mineral in the body. About 80 per cent of this is present in bones, giving rigidity to the skeleton. Phosphorus also plays a part in the release of energy from food and is present in the structure of cell membranes.

### Deficiency
Phosphorus deficiency is very unlikely because it is so widely distributed in foods.

### Sources
As phosphate is a major constituent of all plant and animal cells, it is present in all natural foods. It is also present in many food additives. In general, protein foods (meat, fish, cheese, eggs and milk) and cereals contain more phosphorus than vegetables and fruit.

### Requirements
The Reference Nutrient Intakes are set between 270mg a day for one to three year olds, to 990mg for breast-feeding women. The RNI for adult men and women is 550mg per day. The average UK intake is around 1,200mg per day.

### Achieving the Reference Nutrient Intake
Four slices of bread (300mg), one bowl of breakfast cereal (100mg), 1oz hard cheese (140mg) and a 4oz/113g helping of roast chicken (250mg) or lean roast beef (240mg) will provide the average person's daily needs for phosphorus.

## Magnesium

### Functions
Magnesium is an essential component of all cells and is necessary for the functioning of some of the enzymes which are involved in energy utilisation. It is also involved with calcium in nerve and muscle activity.

## Deficiency
Deficiency signs include nausea, muscle weakness and irritability. Obvious clinical signs of deficiency are uncommon.

## Sources
Magnesium is present in all green plants. The main sources are therefore unmilled cereals and vegetables. More than 80 per cent of the magnesium is lost by removal of the germ and outer layers of cereal grains.

## Requirements
The Reference Nutrient Intakes range from 55mg per day in infancy to 320mg a day for breast-feeding women. The Reference Nutrient Intakes for adult men and women are 300mg and 270mg per day respectively. The average adult intake in the UK is 323mg per day for men and 237mg per day for women. This suggests there may be some minority groups with less than optimal intakes.

## Achieving the Reference Nutrient Intake
300mg of magnesium can be achieved from four slices of wholemeal bread (150mg), one medium jacket potato (50mg), a 3oz/85g helping of spinach (50mg) and a bowl of muesli or wholewheat cereal (50mg).

## Sodium

### Functions
Sodium is the principal regulator of fluid volume outside the body cells, such as in blood. It is also involved with potassium in maintaining an appropriate intracellular fluid environment. Sodium equilibrium is maintained over a wide range of environmental and dietary circumstances.

### Deficiency
Healthy adults can usually maintain balance on very low intakes of sodium, and deficiency is unlikely except in extreme conditions of heavy and persistent sweating, chronic diarrhoea or renal disease.

### Sources
Sodium occurs naturally in food, but the major source of sodium is from salt. Salt (sodium chloride) contains about 40 per cent sodium, the remainder being mostly chloride. In one UK study, only 10 per cent of salt came from the natural salt content of foods, 15 per cent was added in cooking or at table and the remaining 75 per cent came from salt added during food processing.

### Requirements
A safe minimum intake for adults is 575mg a day, and for the majority of

people, the reference intake is 1,600mg. This is far less than the average intake in the UK, where intakes vary considerably but are estimated to be between 2,000mg and 10,000mg a day.

Concern is more frequently voiced about our high intake of sodium, rather than not having enough. This is because high intakes are associated with an increase in some individuals' blood pressure. It is generally accepted that current intakes are needlessly high. Since 75 per cent of our sodium comes from processed food, it would be prudent to return to eating more unrefined, fresh foods.

## Chloride

**Functions**
Chloride is essential in maintaining sodium and potassium balance in body cells.

**Deficiency**
Under normal circumstances, dietary deficiencies of chloride do not occur.

**Sources**
Dietary chloride comes almost entirely from salt (sodium chloride) and sources are essentially the same as for sodium, processed foods being the main source.

**Requirements**
The Reference Nutrient Intakes range from 320mg per day in infancy to 2,500mg per day in adults.

## Potassium

**Functions**
Potassium is present largely in the fluids within the body cells, where its concentration is carefully controlled. It has a complementary action with sodium in cell function. Potassium is necessary for muscle function and the transmission of nerve impulses.

**Deficiency**
Under normal circumstances, dietary deficiency of potassium does not occur. It can occur due to excessive losses, as, for example, through chronic diarrhoea or laxative abuse. Deficiency symptoms include weakness, nausea and apathy.

**Sources**
Potassium is widely distributed in foods, since it is an essential compo-

nent of all living cells. Rich sources include fresh, unprocessed foods, especially fruit, vegetables and fresh meat.

## Requirements
The Reference Nutrient Intakes range from 700mg per day in six to 12 month olds, to 3,500mg per day in adults. The average adult intakes in the UK are 3,187mg and 2,434mg a day for men and women respectively.

## Achieving the Reference Nutrient Intake
3,500mg can be found in a combination of one banana (600mg), an 8oz jacket potato (1,430mg), half a pint of milk (425mg), four slices of brown or wholemeal bread (340mg) and a bowl of wholewheat breakfast cereal (240mg).

## Iron

### Functions
Iron is an essential component of haemoglobin, the colouring matter of the red blood cells. It plays a role in transporting oxygen from the lungs to the tissues and carbon dioxide away from the tissues back to the lungs.

### Deficiency
Iron deficiency is one of the most commonly occurring nutrient deficiencies in both developed and developing countries. The most vulnerable groups to iron deficiency are those experiencing rapid growth, to enable blood volume and muscle tissue to increase, and women during pregnancy and menstruation, especially if experiencing heavy periods. In the Dietary Survey of British Adults, nearly half the women in the study had low iron stores. Iron deficiency ultimately results in anaemia, but even before low haemoglobin levels have been detected, iron deficiency has been associated with adverse effects on work capacity, reduced physical performance and reduced resistance to infection. In children, iron deficiency has been associated with apathy, short attention span and reduced ability to learn.

### Sources
By far the best source of iron is liver. Other sources include kidney, heart, shellfish, lean meat, egg yolks, wholegrain cereals, dried pulses, dried fruit and treacle. We cannot use all food sources of iron with equal efficiency. Animal sources are more readily absorbed than those from plant foods. In spite of Popeye's faith in spinach, it is not a well absorbed source of iron because it combines with oxalic acid, also present in spinach, to form a poorly absorbed compound. Similarly, only half or less of the iron in cereals is available for absorption. Dried fruit, although a

good source, does not contribute greatly to the iron content of most peoples' diet because it is not eaten regularly or in any great quantity. Iron is most readily absorbed from meat, and all iron absorption is enhanced by vitamin C.

## Requirements

Iron is the only nutrient that women (up to menopausal age) require more than men. The Reference Nutrient Intakes range from 1.7mg per day in infancy to 14.8mg per day in women of menstruating age. The Reference Nutrient Intake for adult men is 8.7mg per day. Average intakes of men and women in the UK, from food sources only (i.e. not including supplements) is 13.9 and 10.5mg per day respectively. This suggests that many women may have lower than optimum intakes.

## Achieving the Reference Nutrient Intake

15mg of iron can be found in a 5oz helping of kidney (17mg), a 4oz portion of pig's liver (19mg) or a combination of 5oz lean beef (4.2mg), 4oz pilchards (3mg), a bowl of wholewheat breakfast cereal (3.5mg) and four slices of brown or wholemeal bread (4mg).

## Zinc

### Functions

Zinc is an essential component of several enzyme systems and is part of the structure of all tissues. It is involved directly or indirectly with the utilisation of energy, protein, fat and carbohydrate.

### Deficiency

Inadequate zinc intake can result in retarded growth and defects of rapidly dividing tissues such as skin (delayed wound healing), intestinal mucosa and the immune system. It has been associated with alterations in taste acuity, and zinc supplementation has resulted in improved taste perception. Marginal zinc deficiency is thought not to be uncommon, particularly in the elderly, adolescents because of increased requirements for growth, in premature babies and in alcoholics.

### Sources

Like iron, not all zinc sources are equally available for absorption, and animal sources are the most readily used. The best sources and most easily absorbed are animal foods including red meats, liver, shellfish (especially oysters) and eggs. Other sources include wholegrain cereals and bread and pulses.

### Requirements

The Reference Nutrient Intakes for zinc range from 4mg per day in infancy to 13mg a day for breast-feeding mothers. The RNI for adult men and women is 9.5mg and 7mg a day respectively. Most studies indicate average intakes of 9–12mg per day.

Iron and zinc compete for absorption, and ratios of iron to zinc of 2:1 and 3:1 can result in a significant reduction in zinc uptake. Care should, therefore, be taken in selecting vitamin/mineral supplements which often contain a ratio of more than 3:1 in favour of iron.

### Achieving the Reference Nutrient Intake
Half a dozen oysters will supply you with 27mg of zinc, or you could fulfil your needs with a combination of a 4oz portion of pig's liver (9.3mg) or 5oz lean beef (7.7mg) and four slices of wholemeal bread (3.2mg).

## Iodine

### Functions
Iodine is an integral part of the thyroid hormones. These hormones regulate a number of activities including growth, reproduction, neuro-muscular function and skin and hair growth.

### Deficiency
Lack of iodine in the diet is associated with the enlargement of the thyroid gland in the neck, known as goitre. Infants born to severely deficient mothers are likely to suffer from cretinism. Foods produced in regions where soil is low in iodine, such as the Thames Valley in England and the North West region of the USA, are deficient in this element. Goitre caused by iodine deficiency can be prevented by supplementing the diet with iodine. This is commonly done by adding iodine to table salt, sold as 'iodised' salt. Iodine deficiency is now rare in the UK but is still common in many areas of the world.

### Sources
Iodine occurs in variable amounts in food and water. Seafoods are a particularly rich source. The iodine content of milk and eggs depends on the diet of the animal or fowl, and in vegetables on the iodine content of the soil in which they are grown. In some countries, iodisation of salt is mandatory.

### Requirements
The Reference Nutrient Intakes for iodine range from 50mcg a day in infants to 140mcg a day in adults. Average intakes in the UK are around 245mcg and 175mcg for men and women respectively, according to the Nutritional Survey of British Adults.

## Copper

### Functions
Copper is a component of many enzymes. It is involved in the development and maintenance of heart and skeletal integrity, central nervous system function, red blood cell production and hair pigmentation.

### Deficiency
Copper deficiency has not been reported in humans eating a varied diet. It is stored in the liver in appreciable amounts, so deficiencies would develop slowly.

### Sources
Copper is widely distributed in food. Good sources include liver, kidney, oysters, chocolate, nuts, dried pulses, cereals, dried fruit and meat and poultry.

### Requirements
The Reference Nutrient Intakes range from 0.2mg per day in infancy to 1.5mg in lactation. The RNI for adults is 1.2mg per day. Average intakes for British men and women are around 1.6mg and 1.2mg per day respectively.

## Selenium

### Functions
Selenium is a component of a powerful antioxidant enzyme which protects cell membranes. It is also an essential part of an enzyme which activates the thyroid hormone, which controls the rate at which our bodies use up nutrients.

### Deficiency
No clinical condition has been associated with deficiency. Patients with cancer tend to have lower blood levels of selenium and, along with other extravagant claims, it has been promoted for its possible benefits in preventing cancer. However, there is plenty of selenium in most British foods, and deficiency is very unlikely. Although a small amount is essential, it is a toxic mineral and is not recommended in supplement form without medical advice.

### Sources
Selenium is found in cereals, meat, poultry, fish, milk and egg yolks. The selenium content of foods is dependent on the amount in the soil.

### Requirements
Dietary requirements are not known. High levels (in excess of 1mg) are known to be toxic.

## Molybdenum

### Functions
An essential component of several enzymes.

### Deficiency
Not known in man.

### Sources
Present in commonly consumed foods, such as cereals, vegetables and milk as well as liver.

### Requirements
Requirements are not known, but the estimated intake is between 150–500mg, easily met because of its wide distribution in foods.

## Manganese

### Functions
A constituent of several enzymes.

### Deficiency
No definite deficiency disease has yet been recognised in humans.

### Sources
Wholegrain cereals, fruit and vegetables contain manganese. Protein-rich foods such as meat, fish and dairy products are poor sources.

### Requirements
Requirements are not known, but a safe intake is believed to lie above 1.4mg for adults. Manganese intakes in Britain are estimated at 4.6mg per day.

## Chromium

### Functions
Chromium is an essential trace element directly related to the function of insulin which controls blood sugar levels.

### Deficiency
Clinical deficiency is rare in humans, but marginal deficiency may occur during pregnancy and in the elderly, characterised by impaired glucose tolerance.

## Sources

Liver, brewers' yeast, oysters and potatoes with skins are all high in chromium. Intermediate sources include seafoods, wholegrain cereals, cheese, chicken and meat.

## Requirements

Requirements are not known, but a safe level is believed to be above 25mcg for adults. Average intakes vary from 13–49mcg per day.

## Fluoride

## Functions

Fluoride is present in small but very variable amounts in all soils, water supplies, plants and animals. It has not been shown to be essential to life but seems to play a part in the maintenance of normal bone and tooth structure. Fluoride is known to have a beneficial effect on tooth enamel, protecting against tooth decay, and to make bones more stable and more resistant to degeneration. People with a low intake of fluoride have more dental caries than those with a higher intake. The addition of fluoride to the drinking water has been a major contribution to public health. This has been shown to result in a reduction of tooth decay in children by around 50 per cent. The fluoride content of water is usually described in terms of 'parts per million' (ppm). About 1ppm seems to be an optimal level in drinking water; at 2ppm, mottling of teeth can occur. For maximum effect, adequate fluoride should be available in early years when teeth are forming.

# 3
# FOOD AND
# HEALTH

## — Meat —

Meat has been an important food in man's diet since prehistoric times, yet in recent years it has had a lot of bad press. Rich in protein, fat – especially saturated fat – and cholesterol, all of which are judged to constitute excesses in our modern diet, eating meat is no longer considered a daily necessity for a balanced diet. Protein from animal sources is not essential to human health, as has been demonstrated by the many vegetarians who lead active, healthy lives. However, meat is a rich source of several minerals and vitamins and, when eaten, makes a valuable contribution to our intake of these micronutrients.

Throughout history, humans have generally been omnivorous, not merely carnivorous. This means we have, nutritionally, the best of both worlds. Cereals, fruit and vegetables provide us with some nutrients not found in abundance in foods of animal origin, such as vitamin C and certain B vitamins as well as fibre, while foods of animal origin are more prolific in trace elements and other vitamins, including iron, zinc, copper and vitamin B12.

Meat varies in its degree of tenderness and texture, depending on the site it has come from; muscular sections are tougher because of the coarser muscle fibre and a higher proportion of connective tissue. However, there is little difference in nutritional quality between fillet steak or stewing steak, assuming it is lean.

## Nutritive quality of meat

Most of the valuable minerals and vitamins are in the lean part of the meat (see table below). Although they are invisible, lean meat is also a source of essential, polyunsaturated fatty acids, since they are an integral part of the connective tissue that surrounds the muscle fibres.

|  | Amount (g) | Kcals | Protein (g) | Fat (g) | Iron (mg) | Niacin (mg) | VitB6 (mg) |
|---|---|---|---|---|---|---|---|
| Topside, lean only | 100 | 156 | 29 | 4 | 2.8 | 6.5 | 0.33 |
| Forerib, lean and fat | 100 | 349 | 22 | 29 | 1.9 | 3.9 | 0.24 |

The contrast in nutrient density, i.e. the nutrient content per 100 kilocalories, also contrasts sharply: for instance, lean meat contains 1.8g of iron compared to 0.5g in a fatty joint of meat with the same number of kilocalories.

Beef, lamb, pork and poultry have some different nutritive qualities:

**Beef:** lean beef is a good source of iron and zinc.

**Lamb:** lean lamb is also a fairly good source of zinc, but even lean lamb contains more fat than other meats (8.8g per 100g). This, of course, is reflected in a higher calorie content.

**Pork and bacon:** pork is considerably richer in thiamin (vitamin B1) than other meats and is also a reasonable source of vitamin B6. Pork should be thoroughly cooked to avoid risk of trichinosis, a disease caused by a worm parasite.

**Poultry:** chicken and turkey without skin have the lowest fat content of any domestically reared meat. Removing the skin reduces the fat content by more than half. Duck and goose, in contrast, contain a considerable amount of fat in proportion to protein. Chicken should be thoroughly cooked to avoid risk of salmonella poisoning.

**Offal** (those parts that are removed in the process of preparing the dressed carcase, including liver, kidney, heart and tongue): offal is good nutritional value for money. Liver, for instance, is a concentrated source of iron, copper and zinc and contains considerably more of most B vitamins than muscle tissue. Vitamins A, D and C, not found in other meat, are present in liver and kidney. Liver contains very large amounts of vitamin A which, being a fat-soluble vitamin, is stored in the body. One portion of liver supplies enough vitamin A to satisfy the body's needs for over one month. Because of this very high concentration, the government has recommended that women who are pregnant or thinking of becoming pregnant should avoid liver. Liver, kidney and sweetbreads are rich in cells and therefore contain more nucleic acid than muscle meat. For this reason, gout sufferers are advised to avoid them. Offal is also rich in cholesterol, but if your diet is relatively low in fat, particularly saturated fat, you should be able to enjoy these meats without raising your blood cholesterol.

## Fat content of meat

Wild animals and game, as eaten by our ancestors, contain very little fat because they spend their day actively foraging for foods and escaping danger. The fatty nature of today's animals is associated with domestically reared animals where the emphasis has been on maximising body weight. Intensive feeding methods and lack of exercise help to produce animals far removed from their wild ancestors. Not only are they fatter, the fat is less healthy, saturated fat. Today, approximately 25 per cent of both our fat and saturated fat intake comes from meat and meat products. The fat of ruminants – animals that chew the cud, including cattle and sheep – tend to have a higher proportion of saturated fat than non-ruminants, such as pigs. Chicken has proportionately less saturated fat than beef, lamb or pork.

## Keeping the balance

Since most of us consume too much energy (kilocalories), fat and saturated fat and possibly not enough of a number of micronutrients, the ideal compromise is to eat lean meat. Fat on meat is visible and can therefore be avoided. Lean meat is more expensive per pound, but we could eat smaller quantities. There are plenty of ways to extend meat by adding vegetables, such as kidney beans or root vegetables, or pasta or other cereals, to casseroles, stews and dishes such as spaghetti bolognese. Besides improving the nutritional quality, it makes economic sense in providing satisfying meals without the expense of larger portions of meat.

## Meat and poultry – summary of advice

- Select lean meat – go for quality rather than quantity.
- Trim off visible fat.
- Cook without adding extra fat.
- Grill rather than fry.
- Skim off fat from stews, casseroles, sauces and gravies.
- Use more vegetables in casseroles and stews.
- Skin chicken whenever appropriate.
- Eat less processed meat.

--------------------- **Fish** ---------------------

Approximately 41lb of fish was eaten per person, per year, in the first quarter of this century. By the 1960s and 1970s, that had declined to around 18lb per head, but has since then been gaining in popularity again.

Fish is perceived, correctly, as a 'healthy' food. White fish, such as cod, haddock, plaice and sole, are high in protein, low in fat and a good source of B vitamins and minerals such as iodine and fluorine. Oily fish, such as mackerel, tuna, sardines and salmon, are also high in protein, a good source of B vitamins as well as fat soluble vitamins A and D. They are rich in health-promoting polyunsaturated fats, and where the bones are eaten, as in tinned fish, they are a rich source of calcium.

### Protein

Most fish contain about 20 per cent of their weight as protein. It is a high-quality protein food and, on average, contributes about 5 per cent of the population's protein intake. Because the muscle tissue is softer and is easier to chew than meat, it is considered to be more digestible.

### Fat

The fat in fish is very different from that found in meat or animal products. White fish contains very little fat of any sort (less than 1 per cent of its weight) and hence is relatively low in calories. The benefit of this can be lost if fish is deep fried or coated in a rich creamy sauce (see table below).

In a medium size portion (180g/6oz):

|  | Fat (g) | Kcals |
|---|---|---|
| Plaice, steamed | 3.4 | 167 |
| Plaice, fried in batter | 32.4 | 502 |

Oily fish fluctuate considerably in the amount of fat they contain, depending on the season. They have a high proportion of highly unsaturated fatty acids (from the omega-3 family) which have important nutritional consequences in prevention of heart disease and other diseases. Regular consumption of fish (a fish meal two or three times a week) has been shown to significantly lower the death rate from heart disease. It is thought that this is a consequence of increasing the amount of omega-3 fatty acids, but it could also be partly attributed to reducing saturated fat intake by substituting fish for meat meals.

Shellfish are sometimes criticised because they are high in cholesterol. However, shellfish are low in fat and, as far as blood cholesterol levels are concerned, it is considered more important to have a diet low in saturated fat than in dietary cholesterol.

## Vitamins

White fish is similar in vitamin content to lean beef. It contains, in particular, reasonable amounts of vitamins B6 and B12. Oily fish, as well as containing B vitamins, is a rich source of vitamins A and D. The liver oils of both white and oily fish are very concentrated sources of vitamins A and D.

## Minerals

Fish such as whitebait, and tinned fish including sardines, pilchards and salmon, which have edible bones, are all good sources of calcium and phosphorus. Fish is also rich in iodine. It does contain iron, but to a lesser extent than in meat.

## *Fish – summary of advice*

- Eat more fish of all kinds.
- Try grilling, baking or steaming fish rather than frying.
- Ring the changes by having sardine or tuna (in brine) sandwiches instead of cheese.
- Choose tinned fish in a named oil rather than 'edible' oil (which tells you nothing) or, better still, in tomato sauce.

# —— Dairy products ——

## *Milk*

Cow's milk is the food that would come closest to being able to satisfy all our nutritional requirements, were it not low in iron and vitamins D and E, and high in saturated fat. It contains protein, fat and carbohydrate (as lactose) and is an excellent source of calcium, phosphorus and riboflavin. If you were to have enough semi-skimmed milk to satisfy your calorie requirements (about 4 litres), you would at the same time satisfy your requirements for protein, calcium, phosphorus, zinc, vitamins A, B1, B2, B3, B6, B12, folic acid and vitamin C. Being relatively inexpensive, it is also good nutritional value for money.

There are now a variety of milks to choose from in the supermarket, the main differences being in the fat content, but some also have added vitamins and calcium. Removing the fat from milk, as in reduced fat (half fat) and low fat (almost no fat), does not appreciably alter the vitamin or mineral content, except for the fat-soluble vitamins A and D. Since milk is not a major source of either in our diet, the advantages of cutting down on saturated fat outweigh any loss of vitamins. Milk supplies 20 per cent of the saturated fat in the national diet and, without changing to lower fat milks, it would be difficult to reduce our saturated fat intake to a level in line with current recommendations on healthy eating.

Pasteurised and homogenised milks are both whole milks containing the same amount of fat, i.e. about 4 per cent fat. Homogenised has gone through a further homogenising process to break down and disperse the fat evenly through the milk. It is sold in silver-topped (pasteurised) and red-topped (homogenised) bottles.

Semi-skimmed (reduced fat) milk contains around 1.5–1.8 per cent fat. It tastes less creamy than full fat milk, but most people find it acceptable in tea and coffee. Semi-skimmed milk is not considered suitable for infants under the age of two, since milk may be their main source of calories. Semi-skimmed milk is sold in bottles with red-and-silver-striped tops, as well as labelled cartons.

Skimmed (low fat) milk typically contains 0.1 per cent fat and is very useful in sauces, cakes and soups, if not liked in tea and coffee. Skimmed milk is not suitable for babies and children under the age of five, again because of its low energy content. Skimmed milk is sold in bottles with blue-and-silver-striped tops, as well as labelled cartons.

### When milk is not milk – coffee whiteners

In response to public belief that vegetable fats are healthier than animal fats, a number of coffee whiteners made with vegetable fat are now on the market. To attain that creamy flavour, they are usually quite high in fat, most of which is saturated fat because of the use of hydrogenated vegetable fats. It is, therefore, better to stick to dried skimmed milk instead of these coffee whiteners.

## *Cheese*

The majority of the world's cheeses are made from cow's milk, but they can also be made from goat's milk (e.g. feta), ewe's milk (e.g. Roquefort) and water buffalo's milk (e.g. mozzarella). The milk can be skimmed, semi-skimmed, whole or enriched with cream, all of which determines the fat content. Like milk, cheese is high in protein, calcium and vitamin B2 (riboflavin).

Cheddar cheese consists roughly of 25 per cent protein, 35 per cent fat; the remainder includes water, trace elements and vitamins. In effect, this means that 75 per cent of the calories in Cheddar cheese come from fat. Hard cheeses in general have a higher fat (and calorie) value than soft cheeses, such as Camembert, because they contain less water, the exception, of course, being cream cheese. It is a good idea to read the label and compare the fat contents when choosing which cheese to buy. Choose mature cheeses which have a stronger flavour. You may then need less of them, especially in cooking. The English habit of eating cheese with biscuits or bread and butter or other spread is unhealthy and unnecessary, since around a third of the weight of many cheeses is fat.

Cheeses are generally classified as low, medium and high fat, with cut-off points being below 10 per cent, 10–30 per cent and above 30 per cent fat respectively (see table below).

|  | Kcals | Total fat (g) | Saturated fat (g) |
|---|---|---|---|
| Cream cheese | 439 | 47.4 | 29.7 |
| Stilton | 411 | 35.5 | 22.2 |
| Cheddar | 405 | 34.0 | 21.3 |
| Danish Blue | 347 | 29.6 | 18.5 |
| Edam | 333 | 25.4 | 15.9 |
| Brie | 319 | 26.9 | 16.8 |
| Camembert | 297 | 23.7 | 14.8 |
| Cheddar type (reduced fat) | 261 | 15.0 | 9.4 |
| Fromage frais (plain) | 113 | 7.1 | 4.4 |
| Cottage cheese | 98 | 3.9 | 2.4 |
| Cottage cheese (reduced fat) | 78 | 1.4 | 0.9 |
| Fromage frais (very low fat) | 58 | 0.2 | 0.1 |

Cheese composition per 100g
Data/information from *The Composition of Foods*, 5th ed. (1991) is reproduced with the permission of the Royal Society of Chemistry and the Controller of HMSO.

## Yoghurt

Yoghurt is a fermented milk product made from whole, low fat or skimmed milk. It contains all the nutrients of the milk from which it is made. Low fat yoghurt is a healthy alternative to cream. However, fruit and flavoured yoghurts tend to be high in added sugar. Adding fresh fruit is a healthier way to sweeten it.

Greek-style yoghurts tend to be creamier, having a higher fat content. Some contain about 10 per cent, compared to low fat varieties which have less. That said, Greek yoghurt is still a healthy alternative to cream, which contains 21–48 per cent fat, depending on whether it is single or double.

## Dairy foods – a summary of advice

- Buy skimmed or semi-skimmed milk.
- Only whole, full fat milk should be given to under two year olds.
- Semi-skimmed may be given to children over two years old.
- Skimmed milk can be given to children over five years old.
- Use skimmed milk for cooking.
- Eat more low and medium fat cheeses.
- Use stronger flavoured, mature cheeses for cooking.
- Use yoghurt as an alternative to cream.

## Eggs

The egg stores all the nutrients a developing chick needs, so it is naturally rich in essential nutrients. A hen's egg contains around 80 calories, made up from 7g of protein and 6g of fat. The egg white is made up of protein and small amounts of trace elements and vitamins. The yolk contains half the protein, all the fat and significant amounts of vitamin A, thiamin, riboflavin, B12 and folic acid. It also contains iron, but it is poorly absorbed. The fat in the yolk is generally of superior quality, being largely unsaturated. Egg yolk is a rich source of cholesterol and, when eaten in large amounts, may raise blood cholesterol levels. The general consensus is that it is best to limit the number of eggs to about four a week.

Because of the increased risk of salmonella poisoning from raw and undercooked eggs, it is advisable to avoid recipes which include raw eggs, e.g. mayonnaise, mousse, ice-cream and eggnog or other egg drinks. Eggs should be stored in the fridge.

# — Oils, cooking fats and spreads —

## Oils

Nowadays, there is a wide variety of oils to choose from. The graph on the following page shows the average nutritional content of the more commonly available oils in the UK. Choose an oil that is within your price range, that you like the flavour of and which is high in unsaturates, whether monounsaturated or polyunsaturated (see graph). Get into the habit of comparing the labels for nutrition information. Whatever oil you choose, it will contain the same number of calories – about 135 in every tablespoonful – so it is best to use it sparingly to control both calorie and total fat intake.

## Solid cooking fats

Polyunsaturated margarines are quite successful when making cakes and some biscuits. However, pastries need a harder fat, in which case it is best to choose a solid, sunflower type or one which is low in saturated fat. Again, it is best to compare the nutrition information on the label.

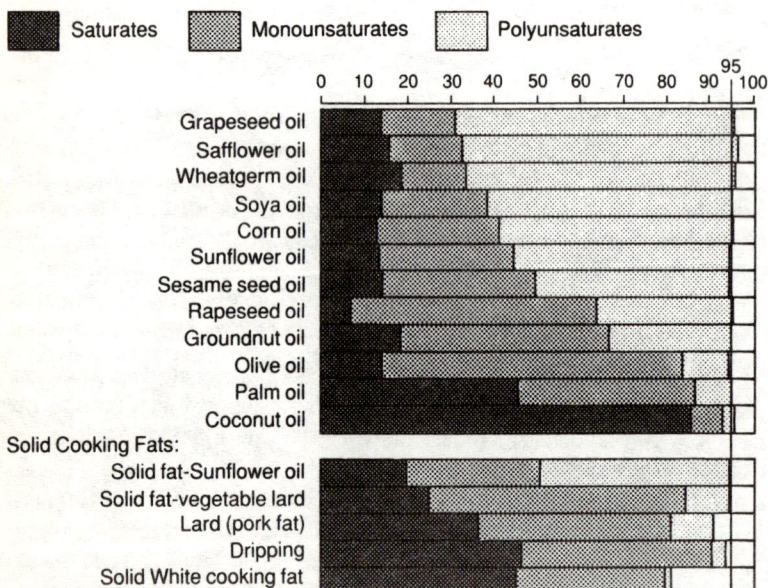

Fatty acid content of the principal oils and fats in g/100g in order of polyunsaturated fat content. (Analysed by the Institute of Brain Chemistry and Human Nutrition)

## Margarines

Once upon a time, there was butter for taste and margarine for cheapness. Today, health is the issue, and it is not easy to unravel the sometimes subtle differences in butter and margarine look-alikes claiming to be healthier alternatives.

Margarine must contain a minimum of 80 per cent fat. The quality of margarine will depend on the type of oil or fat it is made from. It can be made of vegetable or animal fat, but no more than 10 per cent can be cream. It must also be fortified with vitamins A and D.

Choose a margarine that states what oils are used (e.g. sunflower or soya) or at least says 'high in polyunsaturated fat' or 'low in cholesterol'. Currently, the only food labelling regarding fat relates to polyunsaturates and cholesterol. By law, those foods which contain more than 35g of fat per 100g food, such as margarines, which are claimed by their manufacturers to be high in polyunsaturated fats (PUFAs), must contain a minimum of 45 per cent by weight as polyunsaturated and no more than 25 per cent saturated fat. Margarines claiming to be low in cholesterol must contain no more than 0.005 per cent cholesterol by weight. This in itself has little health benefit.

There are two main types of margarines, normally classified as hard and soft. Soft or tub margarines are generally considered more desirable, being higher in PUFAs and therefore better for health. In practice, both types of margarine are made from mixtures of partially hydrogenated and unhydrogenated oils and fats. Hydrogenation is the process by which an oil is changed into a fat, solid at room temperature. It increases the stability of the product by reducing the level of polyunsaturates and increasing the saturated fat content. Hydrogenated oils are, therefore, less healthy than the parent unhydrogenated oil.

In this country, the more commonly used vegetable oils for the more expensive margarines are sunflower and soya oils, but the economy margarines and hard fats may also contain palm oil, heavily hydrogenated fish oils and animal fats. Margarines containing fish oils and animal fat may not, of course, be labelled 'vegetable' margarine. Manufacturers are not obliged, at present, to declare on the label the type or amount of particular oils/fats used in the preparation of margarines. The fatty acid composition of many margarines will vary with time according to availability and market price of oils and fats. The table on the following page gives the average composition and range of various groups of margarines and low fat spreads and of butter.

|  | Total fat (g) | Saturates (g) | Monounsaturates (g) | Polyunsaturates (g) |
|---|---|---|---|---|
| Butter | 80 | 52 | 23 | 2 |
| Margarines 'High in polyunsaturates': | | | | |
| Sunflower | 80 | 15 | 23 | 39 |
| Soya | 80 | 17 | 33 | 27 |
| Oils not specified: | | | | |
| Soft table | 80 | 22 | 39 | 15 |
| Hard cooking | 80 | 29 | 35 | 11 |
| Hard table | 80 | 31 | 39 | 6 |
| Dairy spreads Vegetable oil and dairy fat blend | 75 | 29 | 30 | 13 |
| Low fat spreads | 40 | 9 | 17 | 12 |
| Very low fat spreads | 25 | 5 | 7 | 11 |

Typical fatty acid composition of margarines, spreads and butter per 100g
Analyses by the Institute of Brain Chemistry and Human Nutrition.

## Butter

The battle continues between manufacturers' vested interests in the 'naturalness' of butter and the implied health benefits of 'polyunsaturated' margarines. Butter and conventional margarines have the same amount of fat (80 per cent) the same calorie value (740 kcals per 100g); the difference is in the proportion of saturated and unsaturated fatty acids.

Butter must, by law, contain at least 80 per cent fat, all of which must come from milk fat. This means most (52 per cent) of the fat is saturated. For this reason, it is best to limit the use of butter to treats where it would be missed most.

## Fat spreads

Switching from butter or margarine to a low fat spread can make a significant contribution to lowering fat intake. Currently, no statutory regulations apply to the amount of fat in a low fat spread, and manufacturers are not consistent in their use of terms to describe these spreads.

They use terms such as 'low fat', 'reduced fat', 'light' or 'very low fat', but they can contain anywhere between 5 per cent and 60 per cent fat. It is therefore necessary to check the label for fat content before buying.

Fat spreads can be made of vegetable or animal fat, so can be low or relatively high in saturated fat. Ironically, fats containing less than 35 per cent fat by weight cannot make claims about being low in saturated fat. It is again worth comparing labels for the saturated fat content.

Concern is sometimes voiced about the additives in low fat spreads. It is very difficult to add large amounts of water to fat spreads without having stabilisers to thicken the spread, preservatives to prevent mould growing and colourings to make it look butter-like. However, the likely benefits of reducing fat intake are probably more important than worries about additives.

Low fat spreads are generally unsuitable for cooking purposes because of their high water content.

## Effect of heating on oils and fats

Significant changes occur in edible fats during their exposure to high temperatures. It has been shown that, if fats and oils are heated for very long periods at very high temperatures, the polyunsaturated fatty acids are destroyed and the samples may become toxic. This is unlikely to be a problem with shallow frying, which is normally accomplished quickly, and repeated re-use of the fat or oil is uncommon. Significant deterioration is perhaps most likely to occur in commercial deep-fat frying situations, where the fat is kept hot for long periods with only occasional use for frying and therefore with a relatively low turnover of fat or oil. However, fat which has deteriorated to a level where it may be toxic will no longer be acceptable because of taste and odour. Under good commercial practice, this point is seldom reached, and the fat will have been discarded before reaching that stage.

## Fats and oils – a summary of advice

### Margarine, butter or low fat spread?

Margarine and butter contain the same amount of fat and therefore calories. Butter has a much higher proportion of saturated fat than soft margarines; a sunflower- or soya-based spread is probably the best choice nutritionally, choosing a low fat spread if you want to reduce your fat intake. When choosing a spread, compare the information on the label and choose one with a low saturated fat content.

Choose products appropriately:

**Spreading:** If you want to cut down on fat, then choose a low fat spread, preferably based on a specified oil such as sunflower or soya. Otherwise, choose a soft margarine, again which specifies its base.

**Frying:** Choose an oil that is high in polyunsaturates (see page 64).

**Baking:** Choose a hard fat which claims to be high in polyunsaturates. Compare the information on the label and choose one that has a low saturated fat content.

# Cereals and bread

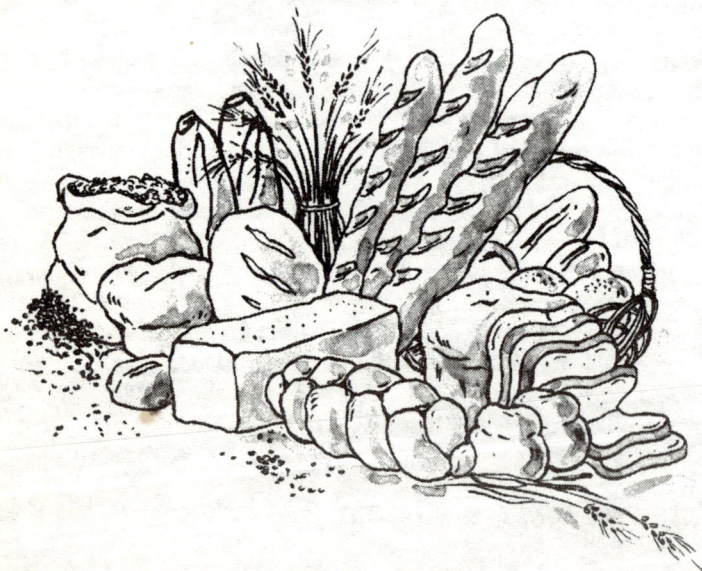

Cereal derives its name from Ceres, the Roman goddess of grains and harvest. Cereal grains have been the staple food of most civilisations throughout the world. The cultivation of cereals meant that primitive hunting communities ended their nomadic life, settled and raised successive cereal crops from cultivated land.

The principal cereals grown today are wheat, rice, maize, millet, oats, barley and rye. Wheat is grown in temperate or dry climates and is the most important cereal in the world, providing more nourishment for the human population than any other single food. Wheat and the breads that are made from it have been considered as the 'staff of life' for many cultures. Rice is grown in damp, tropical climates and is the second most important staple food for man. In many Asian cultures, rice is synonymous with food, yet for most developed countries it is thought of simply as a filler, a starchy base that accompanies meat or fish dishes.

Perhaps one of the most nutritionally detrimental consequences of food processing has been the refinement of cereal grains. Grains as they occur in nature are highly nutritious, but the distribution of nutrients in the grain is not uniform. There are basically three components in the wholewheat grain:

- the outermost protective skin (bran);
- the small area at the base of the grain which sprouts when the grain is planted and is the heart of the grain (the germ);
- the inner starchy section called the endosperm.

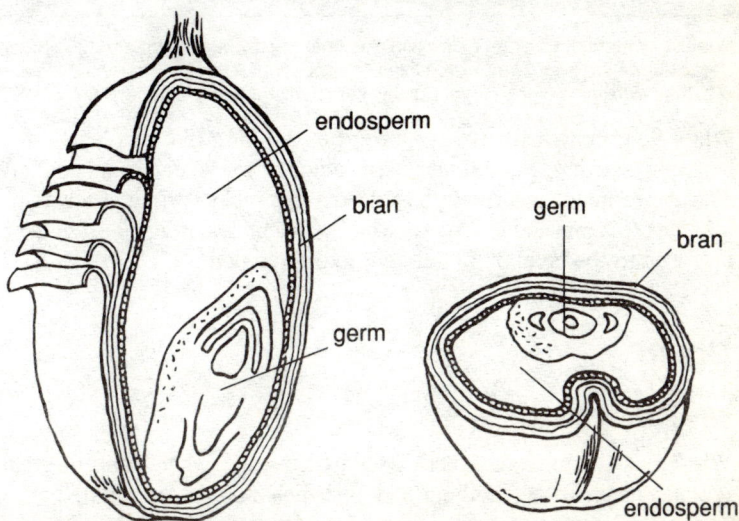

Bran consists mainly of non-absorbable fibre (non-starch polysaccharides). It also contains many of the vitamins in the wholegrain, including most of the B2 (riboflavin), B3 (niacin), B6 (pyridoxine) and B5 (pantothenic acid), a third of the B1 (thiamin), as well as about 20 per cent of the protein. All this is lost when the cereal is refined. The germ contains essential fats and vitamin E, most of the thiamin, as well as smaller amounts of the other B vitamins and 8 per cent of the protein. The germ is often removed from the milled grain because its fat content shortens its shelf life. The endosperm contains mainly carbohydrate in the form of starch, as well as 75 per cent of the protein and some B vitamins. The proportion of the whole grain that is used to make flour is called the extraction rate. For example, an 85 per cent extraction rate flour contains 85 per cent of the grain by weight and 15 per cent is discarded. Different rates of extraction provide different degrees of brownness or whiteness of flour. The table below shows what proportion of the nutrients are typically retained in some common extraction rate flours.

| Flour | Extraction rate | Protein (g) | Fibre (NSP) (g) | Calcium (mg) | B1 (mg) | B2 (mg) | B3 (mg) |
|-------|-----------------|-------------|-----------------|--------------|---------|---------|---------|
| Wholemeal | 100% | 12.7 | 9.0 | 38 | 0.47 | 0.09 | 5.7 |
| Brown | 85% | 12.6 | 6.4 | 20 | 0.30 | 0.07 | 1.7 |
| White | 72% | 9.4 | 3.1 | 15 | 0.10 | 0.03 | 0.7 |

Nutritive content of different extraction rate unfortified wheat flours per 100g/3.5oz Data/information from *The Composition of Foods*, 5th ed. (1991) is reproduced with the permission of the Royal Society of Chemistry and the Controller of HMSO.

White flour contains less than a third of the fibre that wholemeal flour contains (see above table), as well as much fewer vitamins and minerals. The government has made it statutory for millers to put back two B vitamins (thiamin and niacin), as well as calcium and iron. These must be restored to the level of 85 per cent extracted flour.

## Bread

### Wholemeal bread

Wholemeal flour means exactly what it says – the 'whole' meal or grain – nothing taken away, nothing added. Wholemeal bread must, by law, consist of 100 per cent wholemeal flour. It may also contain yeast and water, as well as other permitted ingredients including fat, sugar, salt and 'natural' baking improvers. Wholemeal bread is nutritionally the best choice of bread. Four slices of wholemeal bread a day (125g/4.5oz) will provide 40 per cent of the fibre (NSP) recommended for a healthy diet. However, all breads are good nutritional value, providing you can make up your fibre intake from other sources if you choose to eat white bread (see Appendix 4).

## Brown bread

A wide selection of bread falls into this category. Granary bread recipes vary but have whole, unmilled grains added to the dough. It is usually a medium fibre bread. Wheatmeal bread is usually just another term for brown bread. It is anticipated that this term will be banned by the government because it is meaningless. Wheatgerm bread is usually made from a mixture of white flour with added wheatgerm and bran a certain minimum of fibre. If choosing bread that is labelled, do compare the nutrition information and preferably choose a loaf that is high in fibre. Four slices of brown bread a day will provide 24 per cent of the fibre recommended for a healthy diet.

## White bread

White bread has had a lot of bad press, partly because some loaves, sliced plastic-wrapped in particular, are so tasteless, particularly when compared to some of the more interesting breads now available. White bread is also lower in fibre which, as a nation, we eat too little of, and wholemeal bread is such an easy way to make up that deficit. However, some people do prefer white bread and shouldn't feel guilty about that. Nutritionally, it is not as good value, but it is still much better to fill up on white bread than biscuits or other confectionery. It does contain fibre, but you need to eat three slices of white to get the same amount of fibre as one of wholemeal.

# Breakfast cereals

Breakfast cereals can make an important contribution to both your fibre intake and, because many are fortified, to your vitamin and mineral intakes. A study of New York schoolchildren showed that children who did not eat breakfast cereals but who made up their calories in other ways never made up their vitamin and mineral intakes compared to those children who ate breakfast cereals. Breakfast cereals can, therefore, be a valuable and convenient way of ensuring an adequate supply of micro-nutrients.

Breakfast cereals can vary considerably in both sugar and fibre content, and it is a good idea to read labels and compare both the ingredients and the nutrition information. Firstly, how much sugar is added? It may feature in the ingredient list but not be reported in the nutrition information. Remember, ingredients appear in the order of the amounts they contain. Sugar may also be listed by different sweetening agents such as sucrose, invert sugar, honey, and when listed separately, they can come further down the ingredients list. Next, compare the fibre content; this varies quite considerably from one product to the next. For breakfast cereal manufacturers to claim their products are high or rich in fibre, they should contain more than 6 grams per 100 grams; if they jut claim that they are a source of fibre, then they should provide more than 3 grams per 100 grams.

## Oats

Unlike wheat and rice, the nutritious outer covering of the oat grain is not removed in processing, because oats are not refined. Oats contain appreciable amounts of protein as well as all B vitamins (except B12), vitamin E, iron, copper, zinc and magnesium. Another important nutritional asset is its soluble fibre. The manufacturers of porridge oat products have been quick to make claims about the cholesterol-lowering effects of oats because of this soluble fibre. However, the concensus view is that this is only justified if other components of the diet are in line with healthy eating recommendations, i.e. the diet is low in fat. Bought mueslis do tend to contain appreciable amounts of sugar, so it is better to make your own, using just dried fruit to provide sweetness, and to which you can also add fresh fruit such as bananas, apples or peaches.

## Rice

As with wheat, wholegrain brown rice retains all its original nutrients. However, most of the world's rice is eaten as polished rice, which means it has lost much of its fibre and B vitamins. Polished rice retains less than half its vitamin B6, a third of its niacin (B3), and only 20 per cent of its original thiamin.

| Rice | Fibre (NSP) (g) | Vitamin B1 (mg) | Vitamin B2 (mg) | Vitamin B3 (mg) |
|------|-----------------|-----------------|-----------------|-----------------|
| Brown | 1.9 | 0.59 | 0.07 | 5.3 |
| White | 0.4 | 0.41 | 0.02 | 4.2 |

Nutritive content of brown and white rice per 100g/3.5oz raw weight
Data/information from *The Composition of Foods*, 5th ed. (1991) is reproduced
with the permission of the Royal Society of Chemistry and the Controller of HMSO.

## Pasta

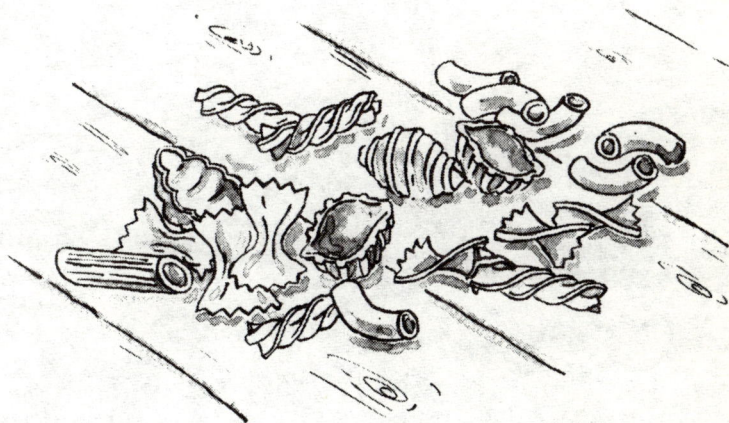

Pasta is made from a hard wheat called durum. Again, the wholewheat
varieties of pasta are much more nutritious than their refined counter-
parts. Like other cereals, pasta is not fattening. The problem arises
when rich fatty or oily sauces are added to them.

| Spaghetti | Fibre (NSP) (g) | Vitamin B1 (mg) | Vitamin B2 (mg) | Vitamin B3 (mg) |
|-----------|-----------------|-----------------|-----------------|-----------------|
| Wholemeal | 8.4 | 0.99 | 0.11 | 6.2 |
| White | 2.9 | 0.22 | 0.03 | 3.1 |

Nutritive content of wholemeal and white spaghetti per 100g/3.5oz raw weight
Data/information from *The Composition of Foods*, 5th ed. (1991) is reproduced
with the permission of the Royal Society of Chemistry and the Controller of HMSO.

## Cereals and bread – summary of advice

- Eat more cereal foods of all kinds, especially wholegrain varieties.
- Eat four to six slices of bread each day.
- Choose wholemeal varieties of bread where possible.
- Spread less butter or margarine on bread.
- Choose wholegrain breakfast cereals.
- Avoid high-sugar breakfast cereals.

## —————— Vegetables and fruit ——————

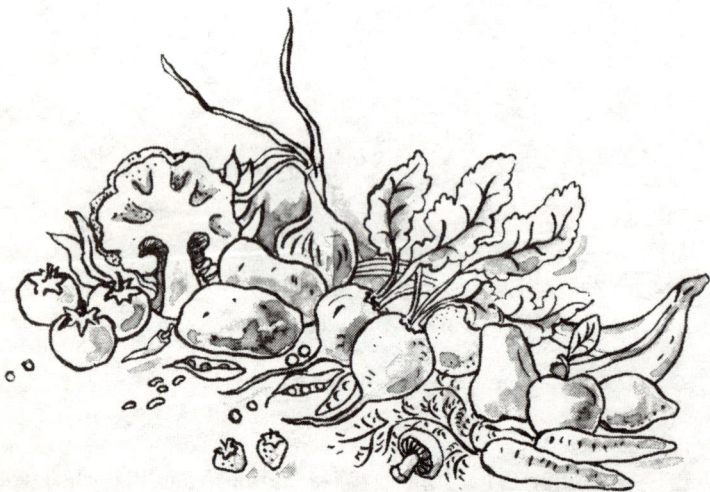

Vegetables and fruit form one of the basic four food groups. They have what nutritionists call a 'high nutrient density' – in other words, for the relatively small number of calories they contain, they have a dispro-portionately high amount of vitamins and minerals.

The US National Research Council Committee on Food and Health recommends eating five or more servings of a combination of vegetables and fruits, especially green and yellow vegetables and citrus fruits. An average serving is equal to half a cup for most fresh or cooked vege-tables, or a medium piece of fresh fruit. It also recommends increasing the amount of starchy foods by eating six or more helpings a day of bread, cereals and legumes, i.e. peas, beans and lentils. These recommendations would mean, for most of us, not just increasing the frequency with which we eat these foods but also increasing portion sizes. Their recommendations are based on studies in various parts of the world which indicate that people who regularly eat a diet high in plant foods have low risks of heart disease and decreased susceptibility to cancers of the lung, stomach and large intestine. The protective effect against heart disease is probably because a diet high in plant foods is generally low in animal fat, which is an established risk factor. The soluble fibre in these foods may also contribute, to a lesser extent, to the lower risk. Vegetables and fruit are also good sources of potassium, which may contribute to reduced risk of stroke.

The way in which fruit and vegetables, especially green and yellow vegetables and citrus fruits, provide protection against some forms of cancer is not well understood, but it is thought to be associated with the antioxidant vitamins (vitamin C, vitamin E) and beta-carotene, the precursor of vitamin A. These foods also contain fibre, but there is no conclusive evidence that it is the fibre itself, rather than the nutritive components, that exerts a protective effect.

## *Vegetables*

The term vegetable covers a wide selection of shapes and biological structures – some are leaves, such as cabbage or lettuce; some are root vegetables, such as potatoes and onions; some are flowers, such as cauliflower and globe artichokes; some are stalks, such as celery and chard; some are seeds, such as peas and beans; and some are fruits, such as aubergines and tomatoes. They also come in a wide variety of sizes and colours. In spite of this variation, they all have in common the same general nutritive qualities: they have a high water content, are low in fat, provide bulk and fibre to our diet and are valuable, low-calorie sources of many vitamins and minerals.

### Green leafy vegetables

These are important because of the contribution they can make to your intake of vitamin C, carotene (vitamin A), folic acid, iron, potassium and other trace elements. The darker outer green leaves are richer in carotene, calcium and iron than the inner white leaves, while the young, tender growing leaves are richest in vitamin C. They are much more nutritious when eaten raw, since cooking will destroy some of the nutrients, particularly vitamin C.

## Flowering vegetables

Broccoli and cauliflower are the two most popular flowering vegetables. Again, because the darker green the vegetable is the higher the nutrient content, broccoli is more nutritious than cauliflower and is a good source of carotene, thiamin, riboflavin, folic acid and vitamin C, as well as iron and phosphorus.

## Potatoes

Potatoes were the staple food of the Inca civilisation about 500 years ago and were introduced to Europe in the sixteenth century providing the poor with a cheap alternative to cereals, especially when the cereal harvest failed.

The potato has a mistaken reputation for being fattening. Eighty per cent of the weight of a potato is water; its energy density is therefore relatively low when eaten without added fat: a 112g (4oz) serving of boiled potato provides about one-quarter the calories (80 kcals) as, for instance, the same weight of roast sirloin of beef (318 kcals).

The table below shows how much the addition of fat makes to the energy content of potatoes cooked in different ways. Frying in oil adds 300 kilocalories to a portion of potatoes. The larger the chip and roast potato size, the less surface area there is to absorb fat and so the lower the calorie value. It is also possible to cut calories with mashed potato by using skimmed milk and possibly a low fat spread or no fat at all. Oven-baked jacket potatoes are excellent until you add butter; why not try a tablespoon of fromage frais instead or, better still, learn to enjoy the delicate flavour of the potato itself without disguising its flavour.

| Method of cooking | Kcals | Fat (g) |
|---|---|---|
| Boiled | 130 | 0.2 |
| Mashed (plus milk and butter) | 187 | 7.7 |
| Roast | 268 | 8.1 |
| Oven chips | 292 | 7.6 |
| Chipped from chip shop | 430 | 22.3 |
| Chipped, frozen, fine cut | 655 | 38.3 |

Energy value of potatoes cooked in different ways per 180g/6oz serving
Data/information from *The Composition of Foods*, 5th ed. (1991) is reproduced with the permission of the Royal Society of Chemistry and the Controller of HMSO.

Potatoes are a useful source of protein, fibre, potassium and vitamins C and B6, partly because of the amount and frequency with which we eat them. The largest concentration of vitamins and trace elements is just below the skin, so they are more nutritious if eaten with the skin or at least cooked in their skin and peeled after cooking.

## Root vegetables

Carrots, turnips, swede and beets are examples of root vegetables, of which the yellow varieties are richest in carotene. They are generally good sources of thiamin (B1).

## Pulses

Edible seeds, including peas, lentils and beans, contain protein, fibre, B vitamins and minerals and, like other vegetables, are low in fat. A cup (170g/6oz) of cooked beans will provide over 25 per cent of your day's requirement of protein, 30 per cent of iron, 35 per cent of thiamin and 10 per cent of riboflavin. They have an added advantage in being cheap and versatile. There are a great variety to choose from, including adzuki, haricot, kidney, broad, butter, soya, black-eyed, chickpeas, pinto and split peas, not forgetting the humble but nutritious baked bean.

# *Fruit*

No other group of foods has such a variety of attractive appearances and delicious flavours. Yet we in Britain eat less fruit than most other European countries. This is perhaps partly due to the fact that fresh fruit does not fit into the structure of most British meals in the way it does in, for example, France or Italy.

Like vegetables, fruit tends to be low in fat and in calories but a reasonable source of protective vitamins and minerals as well as fibre. Avocado pears and olives are two exceptions, being relatively high in fat, largely monounsaturated.

The nutritive value of fruit is perhaps less important than that of vegetables, since the only essential nutrient in which fruit is rich is vitamin C. Citrus fruits, such as oranges, are particularly rich sources, as are guavas, kiwi fruit, blackcurrants and strawberries. Most fruits also contain varying amounts of the B group of vitamins. Yellow fruits, such as mangoes, peaches and apricots, are good sources of carotene, the precursor of vitamin A. Dried fruits are good sources of iron and other trace elements, as well as a number of vitamins, but because, in general, we don't eat large amounts of dried fruit, it does not contribute significantly to the overall nutritive value of our diet.

## Nuts and seeds

Nuts are classified as a dried fruit, consisting of a kernel in a shell. Most nuts and seeds have a high concentration of protein and fat; the exception is the chestnut, which is high in carbohydrate and low in protein and fat. Fat in nuts is largely unsaturated, except for that found in palm and coconuts, which are both high in saturated fat. Almost half the weight of a peanut is fat (see table below), and because they are so high in fat, nuts are also high in calories – ten large peanuts contain about 100 kilocalories, ten walnuts about 250 calories and a tablespoon of sesame seeds, 50 kilocalories. Nuts are a good source of B vitamins and of iron and copper. Seeds are rich in iron, potassium and phosphorus.

| Nut/seed | Kcals | Fat (g) |
|----------|-------|---------|
| Almonds | 612 | 55.8 |
| Brazils | 682 | 68.2 |
| Chestnuts | 170 | 2.7 |
| Peanuts | 564 | 46.1 |
| Walnuts | 688 | 68.5 |
| Sesame seeds | 598 | 58.0 |

Kilocalorie and fat content of some nuts (per 100g/3.5oz)
Data/information from *The Composition of Foods*, 5th ed. (1991) is reproduced with the permission of the Royal Society of Chemistry and the Controller of HMSO.

## *Summary of advice – fruit and vegetables*

- Aim to have a minimum of five portions of fruit and/or vegetables every day.
- Try pulses either as an alternative to meat, or as an 'extender' of meat meals by adding them to casseroles, stews etc.
- Have nuts as an occasional treat if trying to reduce fat and/or calories.

# ——— Conservation of nutrients ———

Regardless of how rich in nutrients a food is when picked, it may not be reflected in what ends up on your plate. The losses subsequent to picking may be due to a number of factors, including the condition when picked, the length of storage time, the way they are prepared, the length of time they are cooked for, the method of cooking and the length of time they are kept warm before eating.

## Buying vegetables and fruit

Choose fresh-looking or frozen produce in preference to tinned products. Freshly picked vegetables and fruit are richer sources of vitamins, minerals and trace elements than those that have been frozen or tinned, since some of these nutrients will inevitably have been lost in processing and storage. However, frozen vegetables and fruit will usually have been harvested in peak condition and prepared and frozen in the minimum of time. They will, therefore, probably be more nourishing than 'fresh' vegetables and fruit that have been stored, possibly in less than optimum conditions, for a few days before being eaten.

Canning requires food to be subjected to very high temperatures which destroys many water-soluble vitamins, i.e. vitamins from the B group and vitamin C. As a result, tinned foods may retain only half (or less) the original content of many vitamins. This exemplifies why it is so difficult to achieve recommended intakes of these nutrients if a person's diet is made up largely of highly processed, refined and tinned foods. As an example, the table below shows the differences that can be expected in the more unstable vitamins in fresh, frozen and tinned vegetables.

| | B1 | B3 | B6 | C |
|---|---|---|---|---|
| | mg per 100g/3.5oz | | | |
| Peas (fresh, raw) | 0.74 | 2.5 | 0.12 | 24 |
| Peas (fresh, boiled) | 0.70 | 1.8 | 0.09 | 16 |
| Peas (frozen, boiled) | 0.26 | 1.6 | 0.09 | 12 |
| Peas (tinned, garden) | 0.09 | 1.2 | 0.06 | 1 |

Vitamin content of peas prepared in different ways
Data/information from *The Composition of Foods*, 5th ed. (1991) is reproduced with the permission of the Royal Society of Chemistry and the Controller of HMSO.

## Storing vegetables

There is little point in buying fresh produce if it is to be stored or cooked in a way that destroys most of its natural goodness.

It is best to shop often for fresh produce rather than storing it for a few days, since this can lead to significant losses of vitamins. Green leafy vegetables should be stored in the fridge in the vegetable drawer. Foods which come in pods, such as peas or broad beans, should be kept in their pods until ready for use. Root vegetables, such as carrots and potatoes, retain their nutrient content best if they are stored in a cool dark place, moist enough to prevent withering.

If you are unable to shop frequently, it is better to choose frozen produce. Foods should be stored in the freezer at −18 degrees C. Even then, as storage time increases, the vitamin C content decreases. Try to use frozen food within three months of purchase.

## Cooking vegetables

To preserve water-soluble vitamins when washing prior to cooking, avoid prolonged soaking or chopping, which allows the vitamins to leach into the water more easily. Cook the vegetables as quickly as possible in the minimum amount of water in a covered pan and serve immediately. If you do want to cut up vegetables or fruit, leave it until you are ready to cook them. Cooking in lots of water for longer than necessary means greater vitamin losses. Frozen vegetables should not be thawed before cooking.

Pressure cooking, steaming, microwaving and stir-frying are all preferable cooking methods to boiling because smaller vitamin losses occur.

Potatoes baked in their jackets retain a higher proportion of vitamin C than boiled potatoes, especially if left whole, since there is less area exposed to the air. Chips, because they cook more quickly than boiled or roast potatoes, also retain more vitamin C.

# Health foods

Health foods are difficult to define, but traditionally, the term applies to products sold in health food shops. These products range from dietary supplements and medicines to normal foods or variations of them (e.g. organic or additive-free) as found in normal retail outlets.

In 1991, a joint working group from the Department of Health and the

Ministry of Agriculture published a report on dietary supplements and health foods (*Dietary Supplements and Health Foods*, MAFF Publications, London (1991)). In its report, the working group was anxious to avoid the term 'health food', since it could be construed as endorsing any implied health claims. It therefore referred to all products as 'dietary supplements' and categorised them into five groups:

1   Isolated, concentrated products such as vitamins and minerals, sold in pill form.
2   Natural substances having known health associations, such as evening primrose oil, fish oils and kelp.
3   Natural materials whose effects may not be fully defined, for example royal jelly, ginseng and herbal teas.
4   Fortified foods, such as breakfast cereals.
5   Slimming aids, including 'very low calorie diet' products and bulking agents.

The working party did not consider it necessary to treat these 'health foods' as different from other foods that make up the UK diet. However, it was concerned that some products, for example comfrey and broom, which had been removed from sale as medicines for safety reasons, may still be sold as foods. It recommended an urgent review on the safety and use of such substances.

It also recommended there should be a maximum amount allowed in a daily dose of those nutrients that are known to have toxic effects when taken in excess. It suggested that excess should be equivalent to one tenth of the 'undesirable dose'. Because the Reference Nutrient Intakes (see Chapter 2, Vitamins and Minerals; see also page 95) for some nutrients does not allow a large margin of safety (e.g. zinc), the maximum amount allowed in supplements may be less than the Reference Nutrient Intake. This was justified, according to the group, because these were intended to be 'supplements' to a normal diet. The suggested maximum daily dose is given on the following page and should be compared with the manufacturer's information when buying a supplement.

|  | Undesirable daily dose | Suggested daily maximum as supplement |
|---|---|---|
| Vitamin A (retinol) mcg | 6,000 | 600 |
| Vitamin A (retinol) during pregnancy mcg | 3,300 | 330 |
| Vitamin D mcg | 50 | 5 |
| Vitamin B6 (pyridoxine) mg | 100 | 10 |
| Vitamin C mg | 6,000 | 600 |
| Vitamin B3 (niacin) mg | 500 | 50 |
| Iron mg | 40 | 4 |
| Copper mg | 30 | 3 |
| Zinc mg | 20 | 2 |
| Selenium mcg | 1,000 | 100 |
| Sodium mg | 8,000 | 800 |
| Cobalt mg | 300 | 30 |
| Chromium mg | 1,000 | 100 |
| Iodine mcg | 1,000 | 100 |
| Flourine mg | 10 | 1 |
| Molybdenum mg | 10 | 1 |

Undesirable daily amounts of vitamins and minerals
*Dietary Supplements and Health Foods*, MAFF (1991). Crown copyright.
Reproduced with the permission of the Controller of HMSO.

The European Commission is expected to make proposals for harmonisation on dietary supplements. If the UK has to fall in line with some other European countries, it could mean that vitamins and minerals would have to be classified as pharmaceutical products if they contain one and a half times the recommended intake. This would, of course, have very serious implications for manufacturers. It is expected that, at a later stage, restrictions may also be placed on the sale of other dietary supplements such as ginseng, royal jelly and some slimming products.

# Organically grown foods – are they healthier?

The term 'organically grown' is misleading since 'organic' means anything that contains carbon, and since all food, whether animal or plant in origin, contains carbon, all food is organic. What is meant by organic farming is a system of growing that avoids the use of synthetic fertilisers, pesticides, herbicides, growth regulators and animal feed additives. Instead, crop rotation, animal or other natural manures, mechanical cultivation and biological pest control are relied on to maintain soil fertility, to supply plant nutrients and to control weeds and pests.

'Organically grown' produce is popularly perceived as being superior in terms of flavour, nutrient content and being free of pesticide residues to produce grown by modern farming techniques. However, there is little good evidence to support these claims except, perhaps, in taste. If there are any differences in flavour, it is more likely to be because of differences in varieties grown, since organically grown produce is more likely to be of an older, more disease-resistant variety which might be identified as 'the way food used to taste' because they were the varieties that used to be grown. A number of blind tastings have been carried out with inconclusive results, although some organically grown vegetables, for example, carrots, tended to be favoured. There is no justification for using organically grown foods on grounds of superior nutritional content.

Organic farming is undoubtedly kinder to the environment. The destructive changes in countryside over the past 20 years or so, the loss of wild flowers, wild animals and insects, such as butterflies, can no doubt be blamed on modern pesticides and other sprays, along with the generally more aggressive farming methods in the use of machinery, removal of hedgerows and loss of woodland.

# 4

## CONTEMPORARY EATING PATTERNS

—————— **Modern food production** ——————

Until 150 years ago, food technology was at a fairly rudimentary level. Methods of preservation were still those used in ancient times – drying, salting, pickling and heating. Food manufacturing and retailing were in an embryonic stage, being small scale and supplying a narrow local market. At that time, food supply was variable and uncertain and relied on seasons.

Since then, the Industrial Revolution has introduced radical changes to methods of food production, processing, storage and distribution. Canning of food started early in the nineteenth century, but domestic and commercial refrigeration have perhaps brought about the most profound changes to food preservation and marketing. Because we are now more highly populated and more urbanised, living long distances from where our food is grown, we are dependent on the food industry to ensure an adequate supply of food to meet our needs. Without the activities of the food industry, modern large cities could not survive and would not have the vast range of foods available to the consumer today. In addition, with increased prosperity, have come new consumer expectations and demands.

Food processing not only allows for protection from potentially harmful organisms, but in some cases, better flavour, cheaper prices and a wider variety of foods to choose from. For example, instead of having peas available for a few short weeks in summer, the consumer may now buy them all year round, choosing between frozen, dried or dehydrated beans or peas in mid-winter, or expensive imported fresh varieties from the Southern Hemisphere during the winter months.

With better transport networks, we now have a much wider choice of foods available and, despite the concept of British conservatism about food, a whole range of 'new' foods is today considered commonplace on our shopping lists. These include such things as yoghurt, rice, pasta, peppers, avocado pears, garlic, olive oil, muesli and ready meals.

Advances in food technology have created improvements in nutritional status; there has been a decline in starvation and in deficiency diseases, an increased resistance to infectious diseases, an increase in childhood growth rates and overall increased life expectancy.

There are, however, negative as well as positive factors in modern food technology. Today more and more food eaten in the UK is processed. When fresh food is processed it usually means that a loss of nutrients occurs, as, for example, when wheat is milled to produce 72 per cent extraction (white) flour. With that process, substantial losses occur in the vitamin, mineral and fibre content of the flour. Losses can also occur by being leached out of plant and animal foods and discarded in cooking water and by being exposed to heat and light. However, these manufacturing losses are often in place of similar losses that can occur at home. The most unstable vitamins are vitamin C, folic acid and thiamin, but losses also occur under particular conditions to vitamins A, B2, B6, B12 and E.

Perhaps more important than nutrient losses is the tendency to make processed foods more calorie dense by the addition of refined sugar and fat. Between 1900 and 1950 world production of sugar increased by nearly 600 per cent, during which time the consumption of starch and fibre has declined considerably. The long-term adverse health effects of these changes in food supply to what is termed an affluent diet is now associated with an increase in a range of chronic non-infectious diseases, including heart disease, various cancers, diabetes, dental caries, gallstones, diseases of the joints and bones as well as obesity.

## Diet and prevention of chronic diseases

A hundred years ago only six out of every ten babies survived to adult life. Such were the ravages of infectious diseases, undernutrition and squalor.

The expectant life span of a man born in England in 1880 was 41 years. Today, this picture has changed radically. Major infectious diseases, such as tuberculosis, no longer pose a major threat to life in this country. Better housing, sanitation, food supplies, medical practice, and so on have improved the quality and span of life to a remarkable extent. Yet today, many are afflicted by avoidable ill health brought about by our affluent lifestyles. Affluence has not proved to be an unqualified bonus. While it has allowed us to largely rid ourselves of many diseases, including those caused by nutritional deficiencies, it has opened the door to others, mainly brought about by overindulgence and undiscerning behaviour. It is estimated, for example, that between 75 and 90 per cent of cancers could be prevented by stopping smoking, changing our eating and drinking habits and improving our environment. About 24 per cent of deaths occur in men and women below the age of 65 years, that is, prematurely.

## Diet-related diseases

In the mid-1960s, evidence started to emerge that diseases not normally associated with malnutrition had their origin in nutrition. In the past 20 years, there has been an upsurge in nutritional research, and the findings are sufficiently convincing for many government committees to call for changes to their national diet.

The US National Research Council has identified eight major chronic diseases associated with inappropriate diet. These include:

| Disease | Main dietary associations |
|---------|---------------------------|
| Coronary heart disease | fat, saturated fat, soluble fibre |
| High blood pressure | salt |
| Obesity | kilocalories |
| Cancers | fat, fibre |
| Osteoporosis | calcium |
| Dental caries | sugar |
| Diabetes | sugar |
| Alcohol-induced liver disease | alcohol |

These diseases are discussed in the next section.

# Dietary recommendations
## for health

Since the publication of the NACNE report (National Advisory Committee on Nutrition Education) in 1983, attention has been focused on the relationship between what we eat and prevention of degenerative diseases. That report was different from many previous reports in that it encompassed the concept of healthy eating in a general sense, rather than dealing with specific issues such as diet and heart disease. It provided a clear statement of a consensus among experts on what constitutes a healthy diet. They suggested that, as a nation, we ate too much fat, saturated fat, sugar and salt and too little fibre, thus increasing our risk of developing certain diseases. The report went on to make quantified recommendations about these nutrients.

Since the NACNE report, there has been a steady flow of publications on healthy eating. The most notable of these are perhaps the World Health Organisation's Technical Report Series 797, *Diet, Nutrition, and the Prevention of Chronic Diseases* (1990); the US National Research Council's *Diet and Health – Implications for Reducing Chronic Disease Risk* (1989) and here in the UK, the Department of Health's Report on Health and Social Subjects 41, *Dietary Reference Values for Food Energy and Nutrients for the United Kingdom* (see page 95). This last report is different from the former two in that it deals not just with dietary recommendations for health and prevention of degenerative diseases but also with recommendations on requirements of kilocalories, protein and essential nutrients, including 13 vitamins and 15 minerals.

## *Do the experts agree?*

It is often argued that the experts cannot agree on what constitutes a healthy diet. The table on the following page shows remarkable consistency between the dietary recommendations of different expert committees.

|                                      | UK 1991 (1) | WHO 1990 (2) | USA 1989 (3) |
|--------------------------------------|:-----------:|:------------:|:------------:|
| Limit fat intake (% kcals)           | 30          | 30           | 30           |
| Limit saturated fat (% kcals)        | 10          | 10           | 10           |
| Limit cholesterol (mg/day)           | No          | 300          | 300          |
| Limit refined sugar (% kcals)        | 10          | 10           | Yes          |
| Limit salt (g/day)                   | Yes         | 6            | 6            |
| Moderate alcohol (% kcals)           | —           | 4            | 30g          |
| Increase fibre (NSP) (g/day)         | 12–24       | 16–24        | Yes          |
| Maintain appropriate body weight     | Yes         | Yes          | Yes          |

General dietary recommendations in different countries

(1) *Dietary Reference Values for Food Energy and Nutrients for the United Kingdom*, Report on Health and Social Subjects 41 (1991).
(2) *Diet, Nutrition, and the Prevention of Chronic Diseases*, World Health Organisation Technical Report Series 797 (1990).
(3) *Diet and Health – Implications for Reducing Chronic Disease Risk*, National Research Council (1989).

## Recommendations in terms of food

### Fat

Too much fat in the diet is associated not just with heart disease but also with some cancers and, because of its high calorie density, with increasing your chances of being overweight. Cutting back on fat, especially saturated fat, should be a priority.

About 21 per cent of our fat comes from milk and milk products, including butter, so being 'dairy wise' is a good starting point in reducing fat intake. There are now many low or reduced fat versions of dairy products:

**Low fat milk:** choose low fat (skimmed) milk for puddings, sauces, on breakfast cereals and in hot drinks. For those who find skimmed milk unpalatable in tea or coffee, choose semi-skimmed milk. This will reduce your fat intake by over 10g a day if you have half a pint a day (5g if you replace it with semi-skimmed). Most of this will be saturated fat.

**Low/medium fat cheese:** check Appendix 3 to see how much fat different cheeses contain. If you eat cheese on a regular basis, you can make substantial savings by opting for the lower fat alternatives. When cooking with Cheddar cheese, choose a mature, strong-flavoured variety so that you can use less of it.

**Low fat spreads:** although not low fat in the strict sense, they generally contain only half the fat of butter or margarine. On four slices of bread a day, this will save you another 10g of fat a day and more if you use it for other purposes. If you choose a sunflower/olive/soya-based low fat spread, you will also be cutting down your saturated fat.

**Fish:** eating more fish automatically reduces meat consumption and has the advantage of replacing saturated fat with beneficial polyunsaturated fats.

**Meat:** almost a quarter of our fat comes from meat and meat products, but you don't have to give up meat to have a healthy diet – simply don't eat the fat. Similarly, by avoiding the skin on chicken, you will reduce your fat intake, since most of the fat is just under the skin.

**Cakes, biscuits, etc.:** a fifth of our fat comes from cakes, biscuits, pastries, puddings and ice-cream, so it is a good idea to consider these as treats rather than everyday foods. Having three good meals a day with plenty of complex carbohydrates, such as cereals, bread, pasta, potatoes and other vegetables, will reduce the need to eat 'occasional foods' such as biscuits.

## Sugar

Intrinsic sugars, that is sugar forming an integral part of the plant cell structure of unprocessed foods such as fruit and vegetables, do not, according to experts, represent a threat to health.

This is not true of sugars not naturally incorporated (extrinsic sugars), and these constitute about 15 to 20 per cent of the average daily kilocalorie intake from food in the UK. There is a lot of debate about the health implications of sugar which may contribute to dental caries, obesity and indirectly to diseases associated with obesity, such as diabetes, raised blood pressure, arterial disease and gallstones.

Sugar does play a part in tooth decay, but it is the number of times a day that the teeth are exposed to sugar rather than the total amount of sugar consumed that is important in dental caries. There is no evidence that sugar *per se* causes obesity. It doesn't matter to the body whether excess calories come from sugar, alcohol, fat or protein; any excess will be stored as body fat. However, sugar is often associated with calorie-dense foods such as chocolate, cakes and biscuits, a high intake of which predisposes to being overweight.

More recently, there has been speculation that sugar is implicated as a cause of disruptive and hyperactive behaviour in children. However, there are no scientific, well-controlled trials to substantiate this suspicion.

Not all sugar is obvious as sugar, since it is added to a bizarre number and range of processed foods. This can, of course, be checked on the ingredient labels. More obvious sources of extrinsic sugar include table sugars, baked goods including cakes, biscuits and pastries, chocolate and sugar confectionery, desserts such as pie fillings, tinned fruit, ice-creams and fruit yoghurts, preserves and soft drinks.

## Salt

High intakes of salt are associated with high blood pressure in susceptible individuals. Since it is difficult to distinguish between those who are susceptible and not susceptible, a population approach in reducing salt intakes is considered favourable.

It is estimated that we consume in the region of 10g salt a day, although there are large individual variations. A substantial reduction in salt intake is, therefore, required to meet recommendations on healthy eating.

Discretionary sources of salt include table and cooking salt, the use of which we can control. However, these sources are estimated to contribute only 15 per cent of our total intake. A further 10 per cent occurs naturally in foods, and the remaining 75 per cent comes from processed and manufactured foods including salted foods such as bacon, ham and other processed meats, a wide variety of tinned foods, bread, breakfast cereals, margarine, butter, cheese, crisps, salted nuts, sauces and pickles.

Clearly, to reduce salt intake means to reduce the amount of processed foods we eat. The food manufacturers themselves can play a role in reducing the amount of salt they add to their products.

## Fibre (non-starch polysaccharides)

A diet high in fibre intake reduces the risk of constipation, diverticulosis and certain forms of cancer. It is also thought to help reduce blood cholesterol levels. Fibre-rich foods are generally less calorie dense and more bulky, promoting a feeling of fullness more quickly than low-fibre foods. For this reason they are a useful aid to a low-calorie diet.

In the last 100 years, fibre intake has reduced by about one-third, and we now need to increase our fibre intake by about that amount. Cereals, especially wholegrain foods, fruit and vegetables are all good sources of fibre. To ensure an adequate fibre intake:

- eat at least four slices of bread a day, preferably wholemeal;
- have a wholegrain cereal for breakfast;
- eat more pulses;
- eat dried fruit in place of sweets and other snack foods;
- eat at least six portions of vegetables and fruit a day.

## A study of dietitians and their families

In 1984, following the publication of the NACNE report, a group of nearly 500 dietitians and their families decided to test how their normal eating patterns measured up to the NACNE recommendations on healthy eating. They kept detailed records of two weeks' food and drink intake; the first week, they followed their normal eating patterns. Their diets were analysed by computer and a report produced which told them which nutrients did not meet the recommendations. They then attempted to change their diets to achieve the NACNE targets. The results of that study, published in *The Great British Diet* by C. Sevekus, I. Cole-Hamilton, K. Gunner, L. Stockley and A. Stanway (Century, 1985), provided many practical lessons on how, without changing our diets radically, we can eat more wisely. The overall changes that they made to their diets to get within the guidelines are set out below.

| Constant but substituted | Increased | Decreased |
|---|---|---|
| Bread | Breakfast cereals | Biscuits |
| Milk | Pasta | Cakes |
| Potatoes | Rice | Puddings |
| Spreading fats | Grain | Cheese |
| Soft drinks | Fish | Eggs |
| | Vegetables | Meat |
| | Pulses | Sugar |
| | Fruit | Confectionery |
| | Nuts | Alcohol |
| | | Cooking fats |
| | | Pickles |
| | | Meat/yeast extracts |

Not only did they increase the fibre content of their diet and cut down on fat, saturated fat, sugar and salt, they also increased their vitamin and mineral intakes because they were eating much more of the nutrient rich foods, such as wholemeal bread, fruit and vegetables.

# — Practical advice on healthy eating —

The first thing to remember is that food is for enjoying and that healthy eating does not mean banning all your favourite foods. Neither does it mean worrying about what to eat or how much more it will cost – healthy eating should not cost more, especially if you are going to exchange expensive, processed ready meals and foods for fresher, unprocessed foods.

Changing to a healthier way of eating should mean making small changes. If you try to tackle changing your diet in a revolutionary way, it probably won't last anyway! You don't have to stop eating any foods, just eat a little less of some and more of others.

No single food provides all the nutrients needed for health, so eating a wide variety of foods is the best way of making sure you get a wide variety of nutrients. There are four basic groups of foods, and if you choose foods every day from these groups, your diet should provide all the essential nutrients you need.

**A   Bread, cereals and potatoes**          four to five portions daily

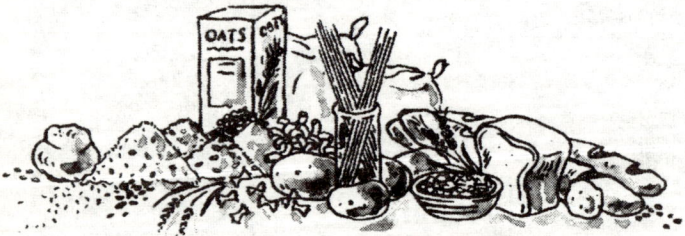

Starchy foods, like potatoes, bread, rice, pasta, breakfast cereals, plantain and yams, should be the main part of most meals and snacks. Choose the wholegrain variety where this is applicable, for example wholemeal bread, brown rice and wholemeal pasta. These contain the

outer germ and husk of the grain and are therefore higher in vitamins and minerals as well as fibre.

It is difficult to get all the nutrients you need in two meals a day. Breakfast provides the opportunity of having a high nutrient meal if you have breakfast cereal and milk, since most breakfast cereals are fortified with vitamins and minerals.

**B Fruit and vegetables** four to five portions daily

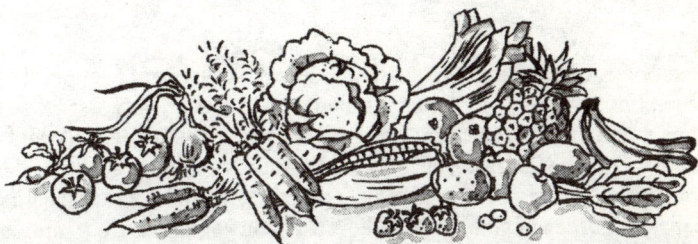

Fresh and frozen vegetables and fruit are all good sources of vitamins, minerals and fibre. They therefore make an important contribution to a healthy diet. Fruit and vegetables are now thought to have a protective effect, helping to prevent certain diseases such as cancer.

We should all aim to eat around 1lb of fruit and/or vegetables every day. This means having at least four or five servings a day. Try to have either some fruit or some vegetables at each meal and snack.

**C Meat, fish and alternatives** two portions daily

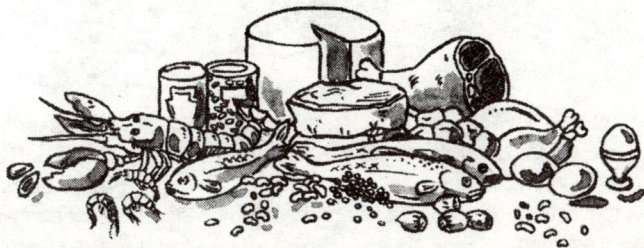

Lean meat, all fish, eggs, pulses such a baked beans, peas, kidney beans and nuts all contain lots of protein, vitamins and minerals.

## D  Milk, cheese and yoghurt        two portions daily

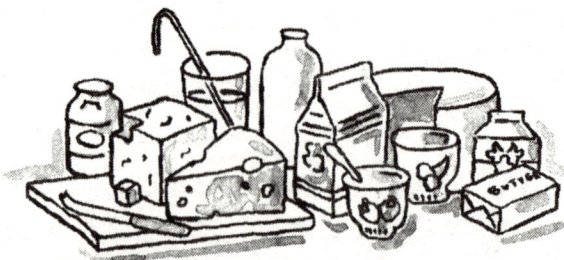

These foods are particularly good sources of calcium and protein. They also contain a variety of vitamins. Low fat and reduced fat versions have just as much or more calcium, protein and B vitamins but less of the fat-soluble vitamins A and D. This may not be important, since sunlight is our main source of vitamin D, and liver, oily fish, egg yolks and margarines are major sources of vitamin A. Yellow fruit and vegetables (e.g. apricots and carrots) also contain lots of carotene, which is a form of vitamin A.

## Occasional foods

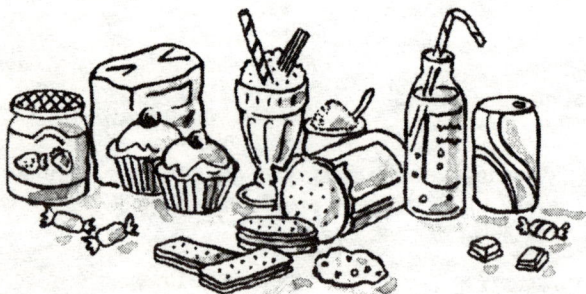

Biscuits, cakes, sweets, chocolates, sugar, jam, pastry, crisps and soft drinks tend to contain lots of calories from fat and sugar and not very many useful vitamins and minerals. They should, therefore, be eaten occasionally rather than regularly and should not take the place of foods from the four main groups above. Butter, margarines, low fat spreads, cooking fats and oils are also high in calories and generally low in essential nutrients, so should be used in moderation. If you use oil and margarine, choose one that is high in polyunsaturates such as sunflower, soya or corn. If you think your fat intake may be too high, choose a low fat spread, preferably sunflower based.

# Reference Nutrient Intakes – what do they mean?

Food supplies and diets often have to be planned. Before information on the nutritional constituents of food was known, dietary requirements were based on the amount of food eaten by healthy people. Ration scales for Roman soldiers was said to be one *librum*, equivalent today to 1lb of wheat per day. Today, we take a more sophisticated approach, and requirements are set not so much by the amount of food we should eat to maintain health, but by the amount of individual nutrients. While this is a more scientific approach, it can sometimes leave the consumer unable to translate this information back into practical information on what and how much of different foods they should eat.

In 1991, a new Department of Health report was published which provides recommendations on energy intakes and about 40 different nutrients. The report is called *Dietary Reference Values for Food Energy and Nutrients for the United Kingdom.*

This report has broken new ground in that the recommendations are not just concerned with requirements for energy and nutrients essential to maintain health and prevention of deficiency diseases, they also make recommendations relating to reducing the risk of chronic diseases through dietary modification. The latter are, with the exception of fibre, more generally to do with our overconsumption of nutrients such as saturated fat, sugar and salt.

New terminology is used in the new report. Previously, recommendations were expressed as Recommended Daily Amounts or RDAs. This was thought by the expert committee to be open to misinterpretation and they elected to express nutrient requirements as Dietary Reference Values. In using the term 'Reference', the panel hoped that users would not interpret any of the figures as recommended or desirable intakes but would use them as a general point of reference rather than as a definitive set of values. Dietary Reference Values (DRVs) is a general term to cover all the following definitions:

1   **Reference Nutrient Intakes (RNI):** this is the amount of protein,

vitamin or mineral that is enough, or more than enough, to cover the needs of 97 per cent of people of similar age and sex. This level of intake is, therefore, higher than many people need, and if an individual is consuming the RNI of a nutrient, they are most unlikely to be deficient in that nutrient.

**2   Estimated Average Requirements (EAR):** this is an estimate of the average requirement or need for kilocalories (energy), protein, vitamins or minerals. About half the population will need more than the EAR, and half less.

**3   Lower Reference Nutrient Intake (LRNI):** this is the amount of a nutrient that is enough to cover the requirements of people with only low needs. Most people will need more than the LRNI, and if they habitually eat less than that amount, they will almost certainly be deficient in that nutrient.

**4   Safe Intake:** this is a term usually used to indicate the intake of a nutrient for which there is not enough information available to estimate requirements. A safe intake is one which is judged to be adequate for most people's needs, but not so large as to cause undesirable effects.

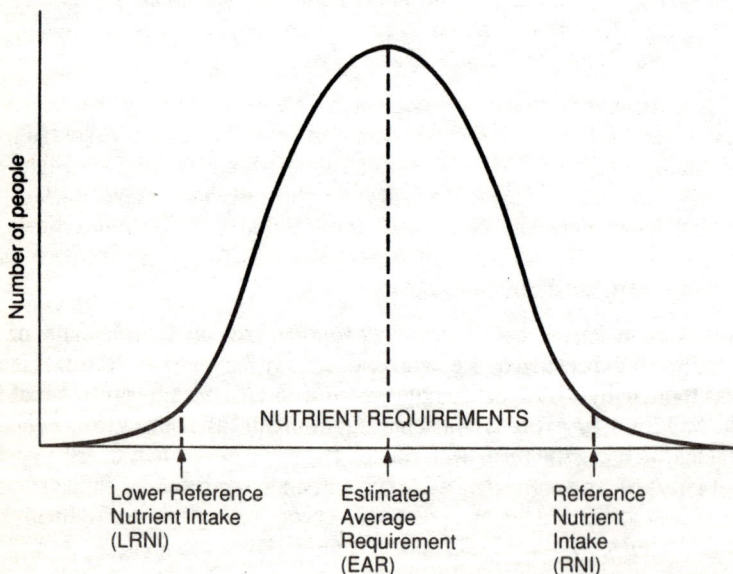

Relationship between LRNIs, EARs and RNIs

## *Use of Dietary Reference Values*

Dietary Reference Values can be used in a number of ways.

### 1  Assessing diets of individuals

Because requirements for energy and for different nutrients vary quite considerably between individuals, even if they all have similar activity levels, Dietary Reference Values have a limited value when considering an individual's nutrient intake and must be interpreted cautiously. If a person's intake is above the Reference Nutrient Intake, then it is very likely that they are consuming enough of that nutrient; if their intake is below the Lower Reference Nutrient Intake, then it is likely that they are not having sufficient to meet their needs. If their intake lies between the two, then the chances of the diet being adequate rise as the intake approaches the Reference Nutrient Intake.

### 2  Assessing diets of groups of individuals

Dietary surveys are often undertaken either by government ministries or by research groups. These can be on a sample of the general population or on different sections of the population such as adolescents, pregnant women or the elderly. It is useful to be able to compare their average intakes with average requirements. Averages do not, of course, guarantee that all individuals are eating enough to satisfy their needs, since some people with low needs may be eating more than they require, and more importantly, some with high requirements may not be eating enough. To ensure that the risk of deficiency within a group is low, their average intake should be at, or close to, the Reference Nutrient Intake.

### 3  Planning food supplies

Authorities planning diets for institutions can assess the adequacy of what they are providing. As with assessing groups of individuals, it is wise to use Reference Nutrient Intakes as a yardstick of adequacy so that the needs of those with high nutrient requirements are catered for, even though this means that more food and nutrients will be supplied than may be necessary to meet the sum of each person's requirements.

Reference Nutrient Intakes can provide a basis for developing national food and agricultural policies. International agencies also use them for calculating food supplies for famine relief and for planning long-term aid to underdeveloped countries or regions.

## 4   Nutrition labelling

Most people will probably be familiar with Dietary Reference Values or recommended intakes in connection with labelling of foods. Here, they can be used to express what proportion of the Reference Nutrient Intake will be provided by 100g, an average serving or a prescribed amount of that food or food supplement. To say that baked beans contain 5.1g of protein per 100g may not indicate to many people whether baked beans are high or low in protein, but to say that an average portion, say 225g/8oz, provides 25 per cent of what a person needs in terms of protein per day, gives the consumer a common denominator which is more easily interpreted.

## *Dietary Reference Values for energy, fat, sugars and starches*

Reference Nutrient Intakes for all nutrients, but not for energy, fat, sugar or starch, are set at the upper end of the range of requirements because an intake moderately in excess of requirements has no adverse effects. For energy, fat, sugar and starch, however, this is not the case, and any appreciable excess intake may result in weight gain over a period of time or may have other detrimental effects on health. Recommendations for these have therefore been set as the average of requirements for any population, and only Estimated Average Requirements have been calculated, not Lower Reference Nutrient Intakes or Reference Nutrient Intakes.

Estimated Average Requirements and Reference Nutrient Intakes for selected nutrients can be seen in Appendices 6 and 7.

# 5

## LIFE'S CYCLE –
———    SPECIAL    ———
## CONSIDERATIONS

___ **Preconceptional care – giving** ___
**your baby the best start to life**

As long ago as 1937, Sir Robert McCarrison, an eminent doctor of that time, expressed the view that 'the satisfaction of nutritional needs in pregnancy begins with the antenatal lives of the mothers [. . .] It must continue during the period of their growth and development up to, during and following the period when they find their fulfilment in motherhood; a fulfilment for which nutrition prepares and makes ready the way.'

This view is still held today, and while it is not possible to change the circumstances of our early lives, many experts are convinced that the way to give a baby the best start to life must be for both parents to be fit and healthy *before* conception. A healthy baby starts with a healthy mother and a healthy father. It is a sobering thought that, in preparing in advance of pregnancy, you may be influencing not only the health of your child but also that of your grandchild.

One of the main reasons why it is important for a woman to prepare in advance of conceiving is that, in the first few weeks of pregnancy, before a mother may even be aware she is pregnant, her baby is developing very rapidly, with cell division at maximum velocity. In the first four weeks, a baby's heart, brain and other organs all begin to form. During the second month, the baby's arms, legs and even toes take shape, the brain grows quickly, and the ears, nose and mouth take shape. During this crucial period, the baby will be relying for its nutrients on what is circulating in its

NUTRITION: AN INTRODUCTION

mother's blood, so it is very important that she has enough to provide for all these developments. The placenta, which takes oxygen and food from mother to baby, begins to form only at the end of the second month.

Of course, no one can guarantee a healthy baby, but it is possible to increase the chances. Preconceptional care, like most preventive medicine, is about reducing risks. The risks of poor pregnancy outcome cannot be reduced to zero but only to a level which is best for a particular couple. Some of the most effective ways to reduce the risks are to:

- eat good food;
- drink alcohol very moderately, if at all;
- be a good weight for pregnancy;
- stop smoking;
- allow at least 12–24 months between pregnancies;
- check any drugs or medicines;
- stop taking oral contraceptives three to four months before conceiving.

## 1   A healthy diet

The aim should be to try and ensure a mother-to-be has ample stores of essential nutrients right from day one of her pregnancy. Every part of our body is made up from the constituents of the food that we eat. This will also be true for the baby, who will rely on the quality of what the mother eats in order to develop and grow while in the womb. For example, protein will be needed to build new tissue; calcium, phosphorus and other minerals for bone formation; iron for new red blood cells; essential fatty acids for development of the nervous system and vitamins to help process all of these nutrients.

A healthy diet is a healthy diet whether a woman is preparing for pregnancy, is pregnant or is simply wanting to avoid heart disease. Advice on healthy eating is set out in practical terms in Chapter 3 (see pages 55–83).

### Liver and vitamin A

The Department of Health has suggested that, because of the very high vitamin A content of liver, it is best to avoid liver if either pregnant or thinking of becoming pregnant. This recommendation has not been met with approval from all nutritionists, since liver is such a valuable source of many other important nutrients. You may prefer to err on the side of caution and avoid it, but a small helping (3oz) once a month will not exceed the undesirable level. Liver is a particularly good source of iron, but other good sources include shellfish, lean meat, egg yolks, wholegrain cereals, dark green vegetables, dried pulses and dried fruit. Iron is absorbed most easily from meat and all iron absorption is helped by vitamin C (oranges, grapefruit, blackcurrants and their juices, strawberries, raw green vegetables and tomatoes).

## 2  Alcohol

Alcohol can damage sperm, so it is wise for the prospective father to drink alcohol moderately or not at all. For the expectant mother, abnormalities have been associated with regular consumption of two standard alcoholic drinks per day or with a massive exposure at any one time (binge drinking), particularly early in pregnancy. As she is unlikely to know she is pregnant for the first few weeks of her pregnancy, it is wise to avoid alcohol or at least keep it down to one alcoholic drink a day when planning to conceive.

## 3  Be a good weight for pregnancy

### If overweight

If seriously overweight, it is best to reduce the weight well in advance of conceiving to allow plenty of time to build up nutrient stores. A government survey of British adults showed that dieters tended to have lower blood levels of some important nutrients. It is therefore important not to restrict food intake either when planning to conceive or during pregnancy.

### If underweight

Some women who are underweight have problems in becoming pregnant, and putting weight on may help them to conceive. Being underweight also increases the risk of having a small baby. It is often more difficult to put weight on than to take weight off, but it is important, if underweight, to make a determined effort to increase it before becoming pregnant. Those who are chronic 'dieters' should stop and allow themselves to indulge in three good meals a day! This will help to ensure they are topping up on all the things the baby will need in those important first few weeks.

## 4 To supplement or not?

If not underweight and eating a varied and nutritious diet, there is probably little advantage in taking vitamin/mineral supplements. However, if taking a supplement reduces anxiety about eating well, there is no reason why a woman should not take one, providing she chooses a good-quality brand multivitamin/mineral which provides not more than 100 per cent of the Dietary Reference Values or recommended intakes for any nutrient (read the label), and that she takes the recommended dose. This is because some vitamins, particularly vitamin A, can be harmful in very high doses (see section on liver).

## 5 Smoking

Smoking harms babies. It decreases the amount of oxygen going to the placenta and the uterus; both are literally life-sources for the baby. A smoker is twice as likely to have a small baby as a non-smoking expectant mother. It is associated with bleeding during pregnancy and with increased risk of miscarriage. Smoking may also be harmful to the father's sperm, so there are very good reasons for both parents to stop smoking before conception.

Giving up smoking is never easy, but is always possible *if you want to* and there can never be a better time to give up than when planning to have a baby. Try to think of the reasons *why* you smoke – maybe to relieve tension, anxiety or cravings or maybe just out of habit? One of the best ways to help yourself stop is to write down the times of day when you smoke and what the cues are that make you want a cigarette. Some people smoke when talking on the telephone, others when writing, reading, watching TV, having a cup of coffee, or when in the presence of another smoker. See if you can change your routine in a way that puts you at less risk of temptation. It is hard to give up smoking, and you may find it useful to contact ASH, 5–11 Mortimer Street, London W1N 7RH. Just think how useful that money you save will be to buy baby things!

## 6 Having babies too close to each other

A baby conceived too soon after the last one can be smaller and less sturdy than their older brother or sister. Having babies close to one another simply runs down a mother's own reserves, and she needs time to build these up again before another pregnancy. Getting fit for another pregnancy takes time. Breast feeding is, of course, recommended for lots of important reasons but, like pregnancy, it does drain a mother's reserves, especially if she is not eating well. It is best to allow at least 12 months between the birth of one baby or, if breast feeding, the time a mother stops breast feeding, and the time she conceives again.

If a woman has a miscarriage or loses a baby, it is very tempting to try again soon afterwards, but it is best to concentrate on getting fit and healthy first.

# 7  Drugs

Drugs, whether legal or illegal, are potentially harmful to an unborn baby. If on medication, it is important to discuss this with the doctor, who may wish to change the drug or moderate the dose in view of the woman's wish to conceive. It is also wise to check with the chemist before buying 'over the counter' drugs for minor ailments.

Hard drugs have the effect of cutting down the flow of blood through the blood vessels. This means the placenta and the uterus don't get enough blood to nourish the baby properly. The outcome is inevitably a small and often sickly baby, less able to resist infection or cope with other illnesses.

# 8  Oral contraception

Some women taking oral contraceptives over a long period of time, particularly if their diets are of marginal or poor quality, may have low levels of vitamin B6, folic acid and zinc. It is generally advised that couples should use alternative methods of contraception for three or four months before trying to conceive.

## In summary

- Eat a healthy diet.
- Stop or drink alcohol very moderately.
- Avoid 'dieting' if planning to have a baby.
- If underweight, try to increase your weight.
- Stop smoking.

- Allow a minimum of 12 months between the birth of one baby and the conception of the next.
- Consult a doctor or chemist before taking medication.

## ———— Diet during pregnancy ————

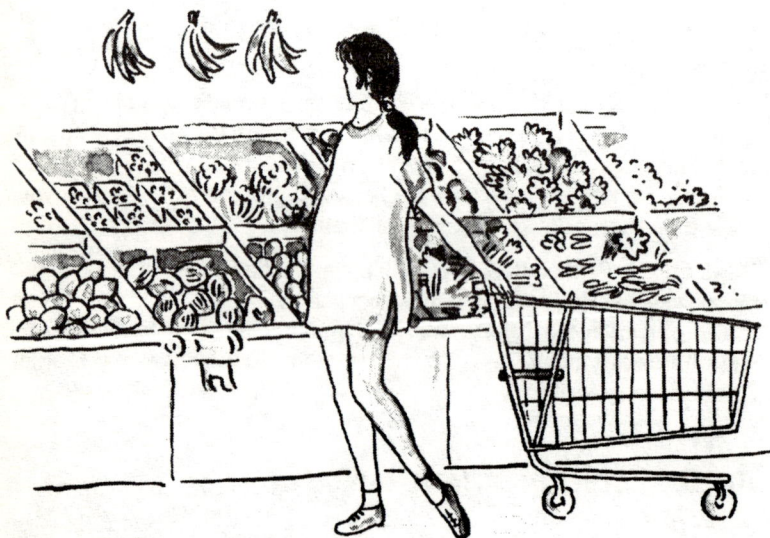

Of all periods in the life cycle, pregnancy is one of the most critical. It is also unique in that at no other time does the well-being of one individual so directly depend on the well-being of another.

Diet during pregnancy is important for both the mother and her baby. The baby is most vulnerable to the quality of the mother's diet during the first three months of pregnancy. During this time, cell division is very fast, and the baby's organs and systems are being established. For at least part of this vulnerable time, the mother-to-be will not even know she has become pregnant. This highlights the need to plan for pregnancy and to ensure a good supply of vitamins and minerals are available via the newly expectant mother for all this crucial activity (see section on preconceptional care, pages 99–104). From the mother's standpoint, a good diet is important to protect her health and to prepare in advance for breast feeding.

Research has shown that those mothers who do not eat well are at higher risk of producing small babies who are more vulnerable to illness. The unborn baby is not a perfect parasite; if it were, it would not be vulnerable to a mother's poor nutritional status. While the placenta is able to concentrate some nutrients to the benefit of the baby, namely some vitamins and essential fatty acids, it is unable to do this with all essential nutrients. It is, therefore, important that a mother has an adequate level of nutrients circulating in her blood, firstly to supply the baby and secondly so that her own reserves are not depleted.

## Eating for two?

While it is important to have an adequate intake of all essential nutrients, it is not necessary to eat for two. A number of changes occur that make women who are pregnant utilise food more efficiently. Absorption of a number of nutrients is increased, calories and protein are used more effectively and as menstrual periods have stopped, iron is conserved for increased blood volume and other purposes.

## Calories

Because of increased efficiency in energy use and possibly reduced energy expenditure, the expert panel on Dietary Reference Values considered it unnecessary to increase energy intake until the last trimester of pregnancy (week 26 to week 40) and then only by 200 kilocalories a day above the normal intake. Examples of what constitutes 200 kilocalories are two Weetabix and a quarter of a pint of semi-skimmed milk; three medium pieces of fresh fruit; 2oz cheddar cheese, two medium slices of bread and margarine/butter.

In practical terms, the best guide to a woman's requirements is probably her rate of weight gain. If it remains within the expected limits, there is no need to adjust energy intake. Attention should instead be focused on the nutrient quality of foods eaten.

## Protein

Traditionally, much emphasis has been placed on the importance of protein during pregnancy because it is central to growth of new tissue. In reality, most people in the UK eat far more high protein foods (meat, fish, cheese, eggs and milk) than is necessary for everyday requirements, even during pregnancy.

## Vitamins

There is a general consensus that the B vitamins should be increased during pregnancy, since they, in particular thiamin, riboflavin and niacin, are involved in energy production. These three B vitamins are found in small amounts in most foods, but only a few are good sources (see Appendix 8).

Folic acid, another B vitamin, has been found to play a very effective role in protecting against neural tube defects, such as spina bifida, when given to women in high doses around the time of conception and early in pregnancy. Folate deficiency anaemia is not uncommon during pregnancy, and foods rich in folic acid should be eaten regularly (see Appendix 8).

## Minerals

Iron is needed for the production of haemoglobin in both the mother and the baby's red blood cells. Maternal iron deficiency in the mother does not normally result in an infant who is anaemic, but it can result in maternal tiredness and make her more susceptible to other sources of physiological stress.

Calcium is important for adequate mineralisation of the baby's bone structure, most of which is acquired in the last trimester when skeletal growth is at its maximum and teeth are being formed.

Low magnesium intakes have been shown to be associated with a higher incidence of low birthweight, and a number of studies have reported benefits from magnesium supplementation during pregnancy. This implies there may be important minorities of women who have low intakes of magnesium.

Zinc deficiency in pregnant animals is known to be harmful and is also thought to be associated with poor pregnancy outcome in humans.

## Alcohol

In the United States, alcoholic drinks now have to carry the warning 'According to the Surgeon General, women should not drink alcoholic beverages during pregnancy because of the risk of birth defects [. . .]'

Alcohol freely crosses the placenta, so the concentration of alcohol in the developing baby will be the same as in the mother. The baby, however, is less efficient at eliminating alcohol and especially so during the first half of the pregnancy.

Because there is concern that alcohol may cause more subtle damage than would be detected at birth, the best advice is probably not to drink any alcohol during pregnancy or at least limit it to no more than one unit on any one day.

## Caffeine

Because massive doses of caffeine have been shown to have harmful effects on pregnant animals, the effect of caffeine from beverages such as Coca Cola, coffee and tea during pregnancy has been the subject of a number of studies. However, there appears to be no convincing evidence that caffeine affects pregnancy outcome. Even so, common sense suggests that pregnant women should have caffeine-containing drinks in moderation.

## Nausea and vomiting

Nausea and vomiting, commonly called morning sickness, usually occur in the morning rather than later in the day and most frequently from about the sixth to ninth week, subsiding around the twelfth to the sixteenth week. A number of factors may contribute to this condition. Some are based on hormone changes that occur early in pregnancy, others may be psychological, based on anxieties about the pregnancy; vitamin deficiencies have also been proposed as an explanation.

Morning sickness can be helped by having a well-ventilated bedroom, free of smoke, and by having a bedtime snack and a dry biscuit or piece of toast before getting up in the morning. Some find the nausea is worse when they are hungry, and eating small snacks every two hours can often provide effective relief.

## Heartburn

Heartburn is generally more common nearer the end of the pregnancy, when pressure from the growing baby can cause acid to be pushed back up from the stomach.

Several smaller meals rather than fewer large meals can bring relief. There are no hard-and-fast rules, but some mothers find fried and spicy foods can cause heartburn and are therefore best avoided. Milk can help by neutralising the acid. Some antacids are safe to take during pregnancy if the heartburn persists, but check with the pharmacist when buying them.

## Weight gain during pregnancy

Desirable weight gain depends to some extent on the woman's pre-pregnancy weight. An extensive study in America has shown that total weight gain for those of normal weight for their height should be about 27lb (12.5kg); underweight women should aim for about 30lb (13.5kg) and overweight women, 15lb (7kg).

## Food safety in pregnancy

Because of the very high levels of vitamin A found in liver, it is thought to be safer not to eat it during pregnancy or if planning to become pregnant (see pages 100–101).

In the interest of avoiding infections from food and animals, the Department of Health has advised pregnant women:

- don't eat ripened soft cheeses (e.g. Brie and Camembert), pâté or partially cooked eggs;
- don't eat raw or undercooked meat;
- don't drink unpasteurised milk;
- make sure you heat cook-chill foods thoroughly;
- wash your hands after handling raw meat and poultry and after coming in contact with any animals.

# - Nutritional needs for breast feeding -

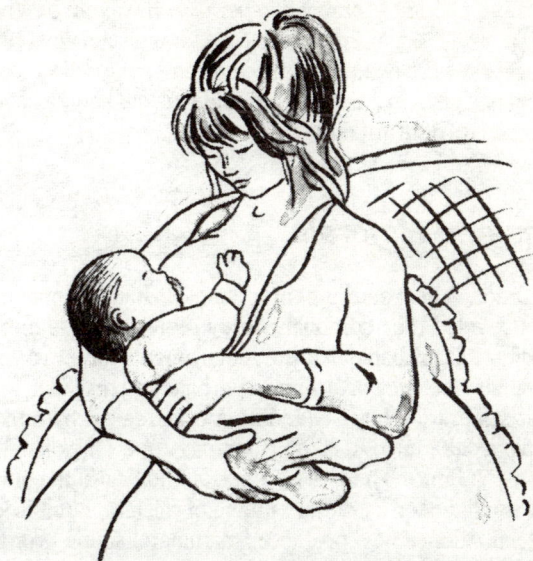

For most women, increased quantities of a normal and varied diet will provide all the energy and nutrients required to produce an adequate volume of breast milk for the baby.

## Energy

During pregnancy, most women build up a store of 2–4kg of body fat as a support for the energy requirements for breast feeding. These requirements are considerable, at an extra 570 kilocalories a day from food sources, along with a proportion of the acquired energy stores built up during pregnancy. A mother's appetite at this time is probably the best guide to her energy requirements. Limiting food intake in order to lose weight while breast feeding is not a good idea, since it may exacerbate any feeling of tiredness and, in severe circumstances, may reduce milk output.

## Protein

Although there is an increment in protein requirements of 11g per day during lactation, making a total of 56g per day, the average woman in the UK has 62g per day, according to the British Adult Survey (1990). If she generally increases the quantity of food she eats, she will almost certainly be increasing her protein intake as well and so is unlikely to have less than the Reference Nutrient Intake.

## Vitamins and Minerals

During lactation, the requirement of most vitamins and minerals is increased. Provided the additional energy requirement is met by means of a varied diet, it is probable that the requirements for extra vitamins and minerals will also be met. Calcium is perhaps of particular importance, since requirements for breast feeding are increased by almost 80 per cent, i.e. from 700mg to 1,250mg per day (one pint of milk contains approximately 700mg). There is no evidence that calcium composition of breast milk is influenced by dietary intake of calcium, but it is known that dietary calcium deficiency promotes demineralisation from bones to maintain calcium levels in milk. It is therefore probable that this may compromise the calcium status of the skeleton, increasing a mother's susceptibility to osteoporosis and bone fractures in later life.

# ———— Infant feeding ————

## Breast feeding

There are a number of decisions that parents have to make about how to feed their baby. The first decision will be whether to breast or bottle feed. Each mammalian species produces milk which is uniquely suitable to support the growth of infants of that species – cows produce milk which is eminently suitable for calves, providing nutrients to ensure quick growth, putting on muscle and extending their bone structure. The human infant, in contrast, has a much slower rate of body growth, not reaching its full physical size until well into the teenage years, but while body growth is slow, the brain and central nervous system develop rapidly and extensively by the time baby is two years old. The constituents of cow's and human milk reflect these differences in development: cow's milk has four times more protein than human milk to support fast muscle growth. Human milk contains much less saturated fat and more essential fatty acids to support the development of the brain, the nervous system and the immune system. Although cow's milk contains more calcium than human milk, calcium is better absorbed by the infant from human milk, and breast-fed babies generally have higher levels of calcium in their blood than those who are bottle fed.

## Colostrum

The milk produced in the first few days after birth is known as colostrum. It provides all the nutrients and water that the baby needs in this early period. It also contains a high concentration of anti-infective agents called immunoglobulins. These anti-infective agents continue to be found in mature human milk but at lower levels.

## Advantages of breast feeding

Breast milk is bacteriologically safe and always fresh. It also contains a variety of antibodies which help protect the baby against infection for most of the first year of life, even if the period of breast feeding is relatively short. This can be particularly important for babies born into less than ideal surroundings, particularly where the opportunity of practising stringent hygiene routines is difficult for the mother. Breast milk costs nothing, it requires no preparation and it promotes close mother–baby contact. Babies fed on their mother's milk are also less likely to be overfed.

Research into intelligence in breast- and bottle-fed babies suggests that breast-fed babies, particularly if born prematurely, have higher IQ levels. It is speculated that the reason for this is that breast milk contains an essential fatty acid called decosahexaenoic acid (DHA), which helps ensure healthy neurological maturation of the brain and central nervous system which develop very rapidly in the last trimester of pregnancy and during the first 18 months after birth. So far, very few infant formulae contain similar levels of DHA to that of breast milk.

Allergy to breast milk is very uncommon, although allergic substances from food eaten by the mother may enter her breast milk. Among the most common foods to cause problems are cow's milk, wheat, eggs and chocolate.

## Problems associated with breast feeding

Of course, there can be inconveniences associated with breast feeding as well as advantages. It is time consuming, and the mother has to be available day and night to feed the baby, especially in the first few weeks when breast feeding is being established. Poor weight gain and an unsettled baby may mean that the milk supply is inadequate, in which case supplementary bottle feeding may be necessary. Breast feeding can create jealousy and resentment with older children in the family. This can generally be overcome by involving them in all other aspects of looking after the baby. There can be a problem in maintaining the milk supply, especially if there is physical discomfort, such as engorged breasts or sore nipples. It can be incompatible with returning to work, but partial breast feeding, for example mornings and evenings, can usually be maintained.

## Formula Milks

Of course, some mothers may be unable to or not wish to breast feed. The common formulae are available in powdered, concentrated or ready-to-feed form. Most infant formula milks available in the United Kingdom are based on cow's milk, but some contain other proteins, for example soyabean protein. Today's formula milks are much better than ten years ago, and advances are constantly being made in getting closer to mimicking the nutritional content of breast milk. However, formula milks still differ nutritionally from breast milk in important ways and cannot supply the antibodies found in breast milk.

In preparing bottle feeds, care should be taken to use once boiled water to make up the formula, to use the recommended amount of powder, to use clean bottles, to sterilise the teats and to check the temperature of the milk before giving it to baby. One advantage of bottle feeding is that the father can enjoy feeding the baby as well as the mother.

If the weather is hot, babies will need extra fluid. Avoid giving them sugary drinks which will encourage a liking for sweet foods and drinks – cooled, boiled water is a better alternative.

## Weaning

Most babies are ready to try semi-solid foods when they are three or four months old. If they do not seem ready to try foods other than breast milk or infant formulae, then there is no need for concern. Breast or formula milks will provide all the nourishment the baby will need up to about six months. By then, they will need to be eating a variety of foods, as well as drinking at least a pint of milk a day.

When starting to wean, puréed or mashed foods, free of lumps, should be introduced slowly, building up the variety of foods. Suitable weaning foods include puréed foods, such as bananas, fish (check for bones), minced meat, potato, carrots, peas, stewed apple and custard, or other cereal-based purées such as rice flakes. If weaning because the baby is hungry, cereal-based foods such as flaked rice will be more satisfying than fruit or vegetable purées. After six to nine months of age, more solid foods can be introduced, such as breakfast cereals (e.g. Weetabix with milk), cheese fingers, bread, plain boiled rice, egg yolk thoroughly cooked, mashed baked beans and pieces of fruit such as banana or apple. By one year, a wide range of tastes and textures should be given so that the baby will grow to enjoy a full range of foods.

## Processed weaning foods

Parents may often feel pressured by advertising in their desire to do the best for their infants: 'If you want your baby to grow big, strong and healthy . . .' The truth is that manufactured foods may occasionally be useful to parents short of time, but they are unlikely to be as healthy as home-cooked food. Many infant foods are nothing like as healthy as they claim to be. For example, some concentrated fruit drinks designed for babies stress their vitamin C content but, for obvious reasons, don't draw attention to their high sugar content. Some baby rusks contain a higher percentage of sugar than digestive biscuits, despite being marketed as 'low sugar'. Clearer labelling both of ingredient lists (see page 20 for list of different sugars) and of sugar content are necessary to enable parents to make the best choice.

# Children

Eating patterns learned at an early age are those most likely to be continued throughout life. However, parents should not allow fussy eating habits to turn mealtimes into a battle ground. Arguments over food can be counterproductive and alienate the child from trying new foods.

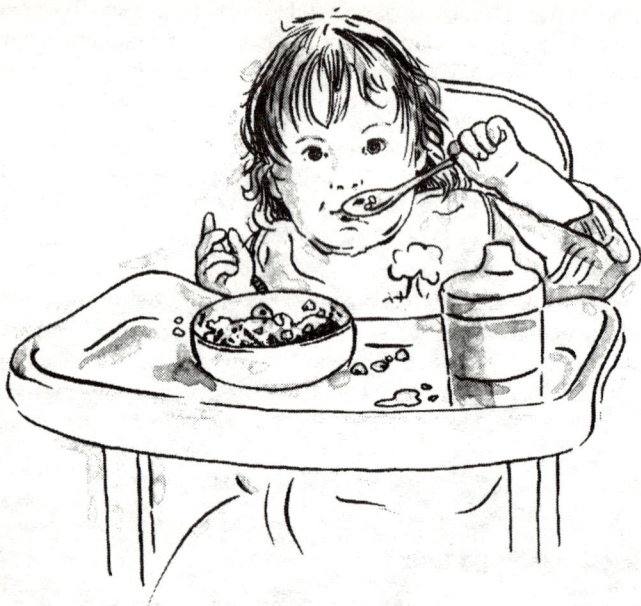

Infants and children are more susceptible to the consequences of poor nutrition than adults because they are still developing and growing. In addition to the nutrients needed to maintain everyday activities, they need nutrients to grow. In relation to body weight, a child's requirements for basic nutrients are greater than an adult's. This means that the calories a child consumes need to be more densely packed with nutrients. There is less room for 'empty calories' in a child's diet.

Small children do not have the capacity to eat large quantities of food at infrequent intervals. It is therefore a good principle to encourage three meals a day routinely and snacks in between, as long as they don't interfere too much with the three main meals.

## Breakfast

Breakfast provides an opportunity for a good nutritional start to the day. If breakfast is omitted, the nutrients that would have been consumed at that time have to be made up later in the day. In an American study, it was found that children who did not eat a cereal for breakfast could make up the calories, but they were unable to make up the vitamins and minerals.

Breakfast cereals are, in general, well fortified with vitamins and minerals and can provide a substantial proportion of the day's requirements, in particular, of the B vitamins as well as protein and calcium from the accompanying milk. It has also been shown that children become careless and inattentive in the late morning if they have skipped breakfast. By prolonging the period without food from the previous evening well into the next day, the consequent fall in blood sugar is likely to increase the drive to snack during the morning on sugary foods.

## Milk

It is generally agreed that children under the age of two should be given whole milk, because they rely so heavily on milk for their kilocalories. The British Dietetic Association recommends that young children under the age of five should drink one pint of milk a day, but from the age of two, providing the child is having sufficient calories from other sources, semi-skimmed milk can be introduced and skimmed milk can be used from the age of five.

## Snack foods

Try to avoid sugary food and drink until mealtimes. It is the frequency with which teeth are exposed to sugar that is instrumental in causing tooth decay rather than the amount of sugar consumed. There are many healthier snack-type foods, including fresh fruit, wholemeal fruit buns, wholemeal peanut butter sandwiches, a bowl of breakfast cereal, wholemeal crackers and cheese, a glass of milk or fruit juice or nuts (for those aged four upwards).

## Packed lunches

Many children take packed lunches to school, and this is an effective way of keeping some control over what children eat at lunchtimes. The basis of a healthy lunch could be:

- sandwich: preferably wholemeal, granary or brown bread or rolls with tuna, chicken, ham or other lean meat, cheese, peanut butter, or egg. Try to add some salad vegetables as well – lettuce, cucumber, pepper or tomato.

- fresh fruit;
- fruit juice such as apple or orange;
- home-made cake, bun or biscuit or small packet of crisps.

Some children enjoy sticks of raw vegetables, such as carrots or celery, which may take the place of chocolate or sweets during break time. In making your own cakes and biscuits, you can control both the amount of sugar and the type of fat used, and hopefully your child will become more discerning about the type of sweet food he or she eats.

## —— Food allergies in children ——

Only a minority of the unpleasant reactions to food are true 'allergic' reactions, where a specific immune response occurs. More correctly, the majority of adverse effects are a form of food intolerance. Discovering which food or foods may provoke intolerance is a difficult task unless the cause is obvious, in which case that food must obviously be avoided. This seems, in theory, fairly straightforward, but in practice it may not be so simple. If, for instance, milk is the culprit, it will become essential not just to avoid milk *per se* but all products that contain milk, such as butter, cheese, cream and yoghurt, or a milk derivative such as casein, whey, non-fat milk solids and skimmed milk powder. These will be found in many commercial products such as ice-cream, milk chocolate, some cakes and biscuits, sauces and many more. Add to this the fact that, for children, milk normally makes a significant contribution to their energy as well as their protein, calcium and riboflavin intakes. A dietitian's help is essential if a parent is to remove milk completely from the diet without compromising their child's nutrient intake.

## —— Diet and behaviour ——

The popular press has paid a lot of attention to claims that certain components of food may be responsible for behavioural changes, especially in children. These claims centre around food additives and hyperactivity, and vitamins and IQ.

## Adverse reactions to food additives

Hyperactivity is a term used to cover a number of behavioural disorders, including restlessness, poor tolerance of frustration, impulsiveness and short attention span.

Food additives are often held responsible for hyperactivity in children. The additives most frequently singled out are the yellow colouring agent, tartrazine, preservatives such as benzoates and antioxidants BHT and BHA (see Food Additives, pages 161–165). While many parents and self-help groups back these claims, there is little scientific evidence to support such cause and effect. Trials are very difficult to do, because behaviour is affected by so many different variables. The Hyperactive Children's Support Group is pioneering work on the link between food and hyperactivity, and no doubt much more will be understood with further research.

## Vitamins and IQ

Following the 1988 BBC TV *QED* documentary on vitamins and IQ, in which children's non-verbal intelligence was reported to have increased following vitamin supplementation, vitamin manufacturers have been very keen to exploit the claims that vitamins are the answer to low IQs. Many new products came on the market with thinly veiled implications of the association between vitamins and intelligence, with names such as 'Top Marks' or even including 'IQ' in the name.

That original study has since been criticised on a number of grounds, not least that the statistical analysis was seriously flawed. A number of other research groups have tried and mostly failed to reproduce the findings so, at the present time, there is no satisfactory evidence that vitamins will boost intelligence levels.

# —— Nutrition and adolescence ——

Teenagers tend more than most to have haphazard eating styles – missed breakfasts, snacking on junk foods, irregular meals and, particularly for girls, crash dieting. They tend to start eating more away from home, so parents have less control over what they eat. It is therefore not

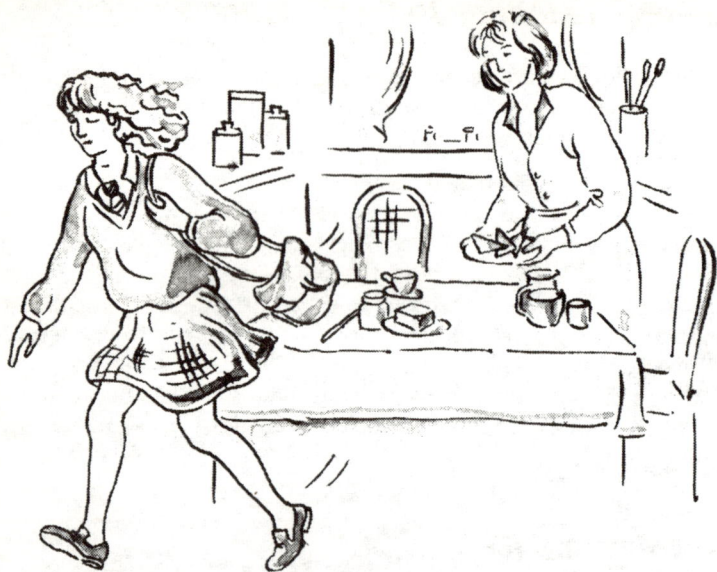

surprising that, in a large survey on what British schoolchildren eat, a quarter of the girls had less than the recommended intake of vitamin B1, 30–40 per cent had low intakes of vitamin B2 and a third of all children had low intakes of vitamin A.

Most children in the UK seem to be able to avoid clinical signs of deficiency, but nutrient shortages may compromise the individual's potential for growth, well-being, vitality and even their ability to learn. During the teen years, calorie and nutrient requirements are greater and, with the exception of infancy, growth is more rapid than at any time of life. During these years of rapid growth, adolescents have been shown to incorporate twice the amount of calcium, iron, zinc and magnesium into their bodies compared with other years.

In girls, the adolescent growth spurt usually begins about two years sooner than in boys, at ten or 11 years, and is usually over by 15. Boys typically start their period of rapid growth at 12 or 13, and this continues until around 19 years of age. Adolescent growth accounts for about 15 per cent of final adult height but contributes to about half of adult weight. Adolescent girls need as much calcium, zinc, iron and most vitamins as boys but they need 20 per cent fewer calories. There is therefore less room for junk food, i.e. high fat/high sugar/low nutrient foods in the teenage girl's diet.

## Summary of advice

Try to make sure you, as a teenager, have the following.

- Three meals a day including breakfast. Breakfast cereals help to ensure a good supply of vitamins and minerals, since they are highly fortified.
- Four or five portions of fruit and vegetables daily.
- At least four slices of bread a day, preferably wholemeal.
- At least half a pint of milk a day, preferably reduced fat. Milk is a good source of protein, calcium, riboflavin and other important nutrients.

If you are worried about your weight and are constantly on and off diets, go and talk it over with your doctor or community dietitian.

# Eating disorders

Anorexia is an eating disorder which is most prevalent in adolescent girls, especially those from the middle classes and of above average intelligence. Sufferers have the ability to avoid eating in spite of being very hungry.

It appears to be brought about by a desire to slim which, for some psychological reason, develops into a distorted obsession with their body shape. In such cases, the underlying psychological problem – the basic fears and anxieties – need to be dealt with as well as encouraging maximum food intake.

Bulimia again predominantly affects women, and sufferers become caught in a cycle of binge-eating and vomiting, sometimes with laxative abuse. As with anorexia, a mixture of both dietary advice and psychotherapy is needed, which aims at restoring a normal eating pattern and reducing feelings of guilt about eating.

It is often more difficult for the underweight person to put weight on than it is for the overweight person to lose weight. Well-planned meals at scheduled hours instead of hastily eaten meals are best. Mealtimes should be periods of leisure and relaxation, since nervous tension is often part of the cause of being underweight.

# Nutrition and the elderly

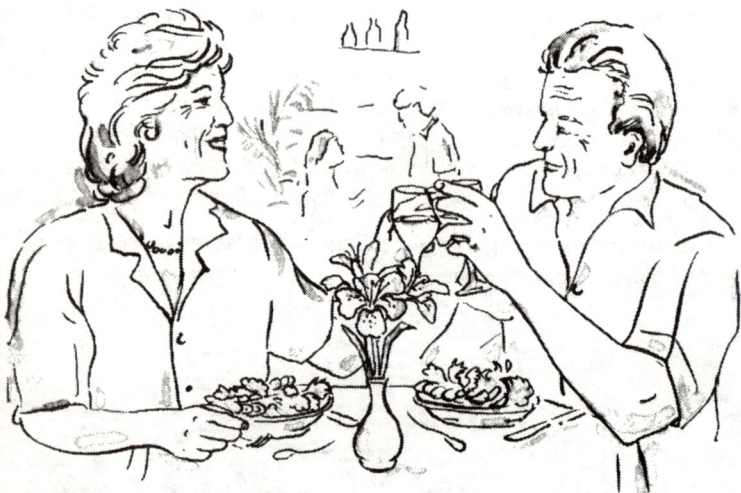

At any age, a poorly nourished person is at greater risk of disease, and is less capable of making a speedy recovery when illness does occur, but this is particularly true of the elderly population.

Today, more people are living longer, and many elderly people enjoy a healthy, active life. Good nutrition can make an important contribution to their health and well-being. Although signs of clinical malnutrition, such as scurvy, are uncommon in the UK elderly population, the influence of sub-clinical or marginal malnutrition on the health of the elderly may be considerable. One of greatest risks for an elderly person is to lose interest in food, and among the most vulnerable are those who have recently been bereaved, are socially isolated or have mental or physical incapacities. These groups in particular may benefit from taking a multivitamin/mineral supplement.

Most peoples' activity levels go down as they get older. Their metabolic rate – the rate at which they use up calories – may also slow down. This means that their calorie requirements also decline. However, requirements for vitamins and minerals do not decline in the same way. In fact, the mechanism for absorption and use of certain nutrients such as calcium, zinc, iron and some B vitamins may become less efficient with age, so there may be an increase in requirements. What this effectively means is that elderly people need less food in order to avoid putting on weight but more nutrients to gain optimum health.

## Vitamin C

Some elderly people have difficulties with chewing and will tend to eat less fibrous foods, like fresh fruit and vegetables, which often contributes to a low vitamin C intake. This can lead to a variety of sub-clinical conditions such as slow wound healing, easy bruising, tiredness and depression.

## Vitamin D

Deficiency of vitamin D may arise from inadequate exposure to sunlight, particularly if housebound, and for such people, a supplement may be a good precautionary measure.

## B Vitamins

A Department of Health Survey of the elderly (1979) identified reduced blood levels of B vitamins in some elderly people, and in some there were clinical signs of deficiency, i.e. sore mouth and tongue, depression and confusion.

## Constipation

Constipation is a common problem for the elderly. A low intake of fibre (non-starch polysaccharides), general physical inactivity, persistent use of laxatives and inadequate fluid intake can all be contributory factors. Regular use of some laxatives can interfere with absorption of the fat-soluble vitamins A, D and E and should be discouraged. The addition of a high-fibre breakfast, such as Weetabix, and changing from white to wholemeal bread, as well as having an adequate amount to drink, will help to relieve the symptoms.

## Fluid intake

Older people often need to be reminded to drink water and other fluids. Dehydration can be a problem for those who don't pay attention to their thirst or who find it difficult to obtain water or other drinks because of immobility. An intake of six to eight glasses of liquid a day is generally recommended.

## Summary of advice

- Try to eat a varied diet; it is very easy to get into a rut when choosing what to eat.
- Have plenty of fibre; wholegrain breakfast cereals and bread will help to combat constipation.
- Drink plenty of liquids.

The overall message is to encourage an interest in food and to enjoy it. Be aware that to neglect one's diet is to neglect one's health.

# 6

## CONTEMPORARY ——— NUTRITION-RELATED ——— HEALTH PROBLEMS

## —————————— **Obesity** ——————————

Approximately one in three adults in British are overweight to some extent, and the numbers are on the increase. Only North America and Australasia have worse records. Over the past forty years, the body fat content of the British adult population has increased by 10 per cent.

Fashion dictates that we should be slim to look good, but our affluent way of life has made it difficult to stay slim. On the one hand, we are surrounded by tempting, ready-made calorie-rich foods that encourage us to overeat, but at the same time, our lives have become increasingly sedentary with the use of labour-saving devices, easy transport and less active leisure-time pursuits like watching TV. In other words, we have less and less opportunity to expend the extra calories that we are tempted to eat through a greater choice of calorie-rich foods in the shops.

Besides the obvious problems of not feeling or looking as good as you could, being constantly overweight can make you more vulnerable to health problems as well as shorten your life expectancy. As your weight creeps up, so too can your blood pressure because your heart has to work that much harder, and this increases your chances of heart disease and strokes. Being overweight can also raise the level of blood fats, including cholesterol. Overweight people have a higher risk of developing maturity onset diabetes, gallstones and certain types of arthritis such as gout, and they may experience more problems with weight-bearing joints.

## *Are you overweight?*

The two most generally accepted ways of telling whether you are overweight or not are:

1. by referring to the chart in Appendix 9;
2. by calculating your 'Body Mass Index' or BMI. This is done by dividing your weight (in kilograms) by your height squared (in metres). Weight in pounds can be converted to kilograms by multiplying pounds (14lb = 1 stone) by 0.4536. Height in inches can be converted to metres by multiplying inches by 0.0254.

Body Mass Index = $kg/m^2$

For example, if you are 63.5kg (10 stone) and 1.65 metres (5ft 5ins), your Body Mass Index would be:

BMI = $63.5/1.65^2$ = 23.3

BMI grades are as follows:

|  |  | *BMI* |
|---|---|---|
| Underweight | = | less than 20 |
| Not overweight | = | 20–24.9 |
| Overweight | = | 25–29.9 |
| Fat | = | 30–39.9 |
| Very fat | = | greater than 40 |

## *Why 'diets' don't work in the long term*

Unfortunately, there is no magical regime that assures easy weight loss or permanent weight control. The fact that so many diet books have made their authors rich and famous is testimony to the failure of all of them to succeed – the Atkins diet, the Mayo clinic diet, the grapefruit diet, the egg and grapefruit diet, the water diet, the macrobiotic diet, the drinking man's diet – all will succeed for some individuals to some extent since they usually limit the calories you can consume and ban high calorie foods. However, many weight-reducing fad 'diets' are nutritionally unbalanced, and some can actually be dangerous; for example, those diets which promote a high egg consumption will bump up blood cholesterol levels substantially; the Atkins low carbohydrate diet is deficient in a number of nutrients which are essential for good health. Perhaps the greatest criticism is that they do very little or nothing to teach individuals how to change their way of eating.

## Very Low Calorie Diets (VLCD)

Very Low Calorie Diets usually contain less than 600 kilocalories a day for a period of days or weeks. Conventional food is replaced by a formula diet. Most of these formula diets are designed to be nutritionally complete except for energy. Concern has been voiced about the efficacy and safety of these diets, which are available over the counter or are sold through agents. In 1987, the Department of Health produced a report on these VLCDs. It recommended that they should only be used when conventional methods for losing weight have failed and should not be used in cases of mild obesity (Body Mass Index of 25 or more; see above). It also recommended that the length of period in which these products are the sole source of nourishment, should not exceed the manufacturers' recommended duration – usually three to four weeks. It pointed out that VLCD are unsuitable for use during pregnancy, for children, for the elderly and also for those suffering from a variety of diseases, such as diabetes. It is wise to consult your doctor before trying these diets.

## A change in your way of thinking about eating

It is important to understand that permanent weight loss cannot be achieved quickly; the extra pounds were not acquired in a few weeks. Give yourself a chance to learn a new way of eating – not to 'diet' as you may have understood it in the past, but to restructure your way of thinking about food in a way that allows you to eat plenty but be more disciplined in your choice of food. This will not only help you shed those excess pounds but will benefit your health in many less obvious ways. Give up the idea of 'dieting' – a diet is something you go on and off. Permanent weight control means a permanent change in both your pattern of eating and in the type of foods you choose to eat; think long term instead of short term.

## Expected weight loss

Excess energy is stored in the body as fat known as adipose tissue. Any weight-loss programme should result in using up these fat stores.

Adipose tissue has a calorie value of 7 kcals per gram or 7,000 kcals per kilogram. In theory, you would have to eat 1,000 kcals per day less than your requirement to achieve a weight loss of 1kg (2.2lb) in seven days.

Normal energy requirements vary very widely from one person to another, but, according to the Department of Health, the estimated average requirement for women, aged 19 to 50, is 1,940 kcals a day, and for men in the same age group, 2,550 kcals. The rate at which you lose weight will, to some extent, depend on what your normal calorie intake has been in the months prior to changing your eating habits.

## Keep a food diary

A group of women at a slimming club were asked why they ate as they did. They gave the following reasons: boredom, comfort, stress, tiredness, habit, availability, anger, to be sociable and, at the bottom of the list, hunger. Can you identify your reasons? The first step in changing any habit is to become aware of it and to know your fattening eating habits.

Before starting your weight-loss programme, keep a diary of everything you eat and drink for a week or so. The exercise of recording all that you eat will pinpoint some of your weaknesses. Do you miss meals? If so, does that allow you to nibble in between meals? Do you overeat when you are depressed, angry, disappointed, bored or emotionally upset? Do you eat to calm yourself or to reward yourself when you have finished the ironing? Do you nibble while watching TV? Do you 'just finish off' the kids' leftovers at teatime and then sit down to an evening meal with your partner? Keeping a food diary will help you to learn a lot about your own eating habits and it may suggest ways you could change your routine to avoid bad eating habits.

## Tackling the problem

There are three main food types that are high in calories but low in essential nutrients: foods high in fat, foods high in refined sugar and alcohol. As a nation, we eat and drink more of these than is good for our health, whether overweight or not. Reducing the amount of these will automatically reduce calorie intakes. In cases where weight is not a problem, these calories should be replaced with starchy foods, also known as complex carbohydrates, such as wholemeal bread and cereals, pasta, rice and potatoes. Where there is a need to lose weight, it may be necessary to restrict these and other calorie-containing foods, depending on the normal contribution fat, sugar and alcohol make to your calorie intake and how much you are willing to cut them down.

## Fat

Fat is the most concentrated source of calories in our diet, so must be restricted if calories are to be reduced. Fat contains 9 calories for every gram, so 1 teaspoon (5ml) of oil contains 40 calories – about the same as in a medium-sized apple. Not all fats are as obvious as oil, margarine or butter. Less evident sources of fat include dairy produce (cheese, milk, cream and made-up dishes containing them), meat and meat products, poultry skin, eggs, nuts, seeds and foods made with fat or oil such as biscuits, cakes, pastry, crisps, chocolate, salad creams, dressings and mayonnaise.

## Sugar

Sugar and high-sugar foods should also be on the hit list! While sugar is not so calorie dense as fat, high-sugar foods are generally 'poor value for calories' because they provide you with calories and very little else in the way of vitamins and minerals. Additionally, high-sugar foods are often also high in fat and therefore high in calories: biscuits, cakes, puddings and confectionery such as chocolates and toffees all come under this category. High-sugar foods include white and brown sugar, golden syrup, honey, jam, marmalade, sweets, chocolates, fruit tinned in syrup or any foods or drinks sweetened with sugar, sucrose, glucose, fructose, dextrose and syrups (look at the labels).

## Alcohol

Alcohol is high in calories, low in essential vitamins and minerals and should not really be included in a weight-reducing plan. In terms of a pub measure, the lowest calorie choice of alcoholic drinks would be a tot of spirit (50 kcals) with a low-calorie mixer or a measure of dry vermouth (55 kcals).

## Non-starch polysaccharides: fibre

Foods containing fibre are filling because they are bulky, but not fattening because they are generally low in fat. A diet high in fibre is generally a good indication of a high vitamin and mineral intake, since high-fibre foods are associated with lots of vitamins and minerals; for example, fruit and vegetables are both high in fibre and a good source of essential vitamins;

wholegrain cereals are also much more nutritious than refined cereals which have had the husk removed, because the fibre and most of the nutrients are concentrated around the outside of the grain, the husk. Fruit and vegetables (with the exception of avocado pears and olives) have the added advantage of being relatively low in calories, since they have a minimal fat content and a high water content, providing bulk to satisfy your appetite but with few calories. For example, five pieces of fresh fruit, such as five apples or five oranges, have approximately the same number of calories as a 56g/2oz bar of chocolate or a 2oz packet of peanuts, and the fruit would also supply a lot more essential vitamins as well.

Remember, if you go off the rails once or twice, don't let that serve as an excuse to give up. The approach to aim for is to change your long-term eating habits to a healthier way of eating which will benefit all the family. If you reduce your fat, sugar and alcohol intake even by half your normal intake, you will lose weight. The loss may not be dramatically quick, but your new, healthier way of eating will help you to keep those unwanted pounds off.

## Three meals a day

A very important strategy is to learn to have three meals a day. This helps to reduce the temptation to nibble high-calorie snacks between meals. If you're not especially hungry for one of the meals, eat less, but always eat something and never skip breakfast, lunch or the evening meal.

### Breakfast

The habit of skipping breakfast can be hard to break, but do persevere. Be adventurous – it need not be a plate of cereal and low fat milk every morning. Try some of the delicious fruits in season, maybe mango or kiwi fruit, strawberries or melon, guava or peaches, sharon fruit or apricots. Don't be afraid to try new fruits. In the winter, try stewed, fresh or dried fruits, such as pears or apples, with plain yoghurt or low fat fromage frais. If you like breakfast cereals, choose a high fibre type such as Shredded Wheat or Weetabix. When buying cereals, look at the label and compare the fibre content. In the winter, you may like to ring the changes with porridge made with low fat milk, or grilled tomatoes or mushrooms cooked with a little lemon juice on wholemeal toast and low fat spread used very sparingly.

## Lunch

Many of us rely on sandwiches or rolls for lunch. It is much easier to control the calories if you make your own: you can use low fat spread (or none) instead of margarine or butter, choose low or medium fat cheese such as Edam, Brie or curd instead of full fat cheeses, omit mayonnaises and enhance the filling with lots of salad vegetables such as peppers or watercress. Choose wholemeal bread in preference to white and don't forget some fresh fruit. If you are at home during the day, you may like to make a good vegetable soup or stew with lots of fresh vegetables in season or perhaps baked beans on wholemeal toast or a large bowl of fresh fruit salad with fromage frais.

## Evening meal

As long as you are prepared to choose foods which are not high in fat or in sugar, you should be in a position to eat well without overdoing the calories. Choose lean cuts of meat or, better still, white fish which is very low in fat (but avoid adding fat in cooking). Fill up on vegetables, salads and potatoes, rice or pasta, preferably brown or wholewheat. Contrary to popular belief, these starchy foods are not high in calories and will help to satisfy your appetite.

## Eating out

It is usually possible to make a suitable choice when eating out, without feeling too deprived. For example, your starter could be melon, with or without lean Parma ham, grapefruit, consommé, oysters or smoked salmon. For the main course choose lean grilled meat or liver, grilled fish or any sea food served without sauces, boiled or jacket potato and any vegetable not cooked in or served with fat, butter or cream, or salad without dressing. For dessert, any fresh fruit, for example strawberries, fresh figs or fresh fruit salad, would be ideal, so long as no cream is added. Do ask whoever you are eating out with for their support and not to try to tempt you into making the wrong choices. If you are having a glass of wine, try having half wine and half carbonated mineral water: that way you get two for the price of one glass!

## Exercise

Exercise must be an important component of any weight-loss programme. Increased physical activity has several benefits. Weight loss by calorie restriction without exercise typically comes from a 75 per cent loss of fat and 25 per cent loss of muscle. By exercising regularly during calorie restriction, the amount of muscle loss can be reduced to only 5 per cent. Exercise also speeds up metabolic rate, lowers blood pressure, decreases blood lipids (fats); it increases stamina and improves self-esteem. Try to aim at some form of physical exertion for a minimum of 30 minutes three times a week. Choose a form of exercise that you enjoy such as brisk walking, bike-riding, dancing, aerobics or swimming. If you have an hour for lunch, why not use half an hour for your lunch and the other half for a brisk walk or jog?

## Weight maintenance

Once you have achieved your target weight, that is a Body Mass Index of 20 to 25, then you can increase the amount of food that you eat, but try to keep your intake of fat, refined sugar and alcohol under control. Keep a regular check on your weight and if it does start to creep up, try to identify the reasons for it and act on them.

## Slenderising ways!

- Eat three meals a day – no snacking in between!
- Eat more slowly. Put less food on your fork at a time, chew your food for longer and put your utensils down between each mouthful.
- Serve yourself on a smaller plate – you will feel less deprived by skimpy servings.
- Restrict all your eating to one or two appropriate places in your home – for example, the kitchen and dining room tables – and sit down to eat at those places. No eating in the car or at your desk.
- Go grocery shopping after you have eaten, not when you are feeling hungry. Make a detailed shopping list and stick to it.
- Avoid buying your problem foods.
- Get someone else in the family to clear the plates and put away the leftovers.
- If certain activities are associated with in-between-meal eating, change your routine.
- Let your family and friends know that you are trying to cut down. Tell them that the most caring thing they can do for you is not offer you anything to eat.
- Slimming with someone else can be easier.

# ———— Coronary heart disease ————

Almost half the deaths in England and Wales are caused by some form of circulatory disease. It is the biggest single cause of death in the UK. Although most of the deaths occur over the age of 65, it is the leading cause of premature death in men and comes second only to cancer as the main cause of premature death in women.

Yet, in spite of the social and economic devastation that heart disease can cause, most experts agree that it is largely preventable because its occurrence is strongly associated with the way we live. Smoking, poor diet, physical inactivity and obesity are all 'modifiable' risk factors. We as individuals can help to reduce our own risk of heart disease and other diseases associated with our modern lifestyle.

## *Atherosclerosis – the heart of the problem*

At the centre of the problem is a disease called atherosclerosis, which is a combination of changes that occur in the inner lining of arteries, resulting in localised accumulation of fatty deposits in the artery wall. These deposits consist mainly of cell debris and a fatty substance called cholesterol. The process of atherosclerosis can also lead to loss of elasticity of arteries, so that they become more rigid or 'hardened', and so further reduce the efficiency of blood circulation. The deposits gradually reduce the blood vessels' diameter and, as the arteries become narrower, the flow of blood to the heart becomes increasingly restricted. This can cause quite severe chest pain (angina), especially following some form of exertion or excitement which requires an increase in oxygen, and therefore blood flow, to the heart. If an artery becomes so furred up or narrowed that it blocks the flow of blood to the heart completely, a heart attack occurs. A heart attack can also occur if a circulating blood clot closes an already narrowed artery; this is called a coronary thrombosis.

There is a fine balance between the ability of blood to clot or 'thrombose' in response to injury and maintaining a normal blood flow through healthy blood vessels. If blood clots quickly, it is beneficial in that it prevents excessive blood loss when injury occurs, but it also means there is an increased risk of developing blood clots which may lead to a heart attack.

Diet plays an important part both in the regulation of blood cholesterol levels and the mechanism regulating blood clotting.

# What are the risk factors associated with heart disease?

A number of risk factors have been identified and have been shown to be strongly associated with the development of heart disease. Some of these factors cannot be altered, for example being male, growing old or having a family history of heart disease, but many, and possibly the most important, risk factors are within our own power to control by a change in lifestyle and eating habits. Cigarette smoking, high blood pressure and high blood fat levels are the most clearly established of these factors, but lack of exercise, being overweight, suffering from diabetes and stress are also thought to be associated. All of these, separately and in combination, foster the risk of illness and premature death from heart disease.

# Expert reports and recommendations

In the past few years, many expert committees, both in the UK and internationally, have published recommendations on healthy eating. Some recommendations have dealt specifically with prevention of heart disease, while others have considered healthy eating in terms of prevention of all diet-related illnesses. In any event, the recommendations are very similar; all, without exception, have recommended that we lower our total fat intake from a current national average 42 per cent of our calories to no more than 30 to 35 per cent, and our saturated fat should be reduced from 17 to 10 per cent of our energy intake. That means cutting total fat by about a quarter and cutting saturated fat by almost a half.

It is also recommended that fibre should be increased by 50 per cent, that is from 20g a day to 30g a day, and we should restrict our consumption of added (extrinsic) sugar and salt.

## Fats in blood

The two most important fats circulating in blood are cholesterol and triglycerides. Raised blood levels of either of these components are potential risk factors of heart disease.

# Cholesterol confusion?

## Blood cholesterol

Cholesterol is an essential part of cell membranes. It is also necessary for moulding the casing that protects nerve fibres and to help produce vitamin D and certain hormones, including the sex hormones.

Cholesterol in the blood comes from two sources. The main source is endogenous production, i.e. made within the body, mainly by the liver. The second source is from cholesterol in the food we eat. The cholesterol level in blood is influenced much more by the type and amount of fat in your diet than the amount of cholesterol in your diet. If a healthy individual decreases the amount of cholesterol in their diet, the rate of absorption is increased and, conversely, if they were to increase their cholesterol intake, the rate of absorption is decreased. As a result, dietary modification of cholesterol does not have a large impact on blood cholesterol levels. However, a high cholesterol intake can raise blood cholesterol levels, and if you do have a high blood cholesterol, it is prudent not to exacerbate the problem by eating a lot of cholesterol-rich foods.

| Blood cholesterol level | Risk of heart disease |
| --- | --- |
| Less than 5.2mmol per litre | Low |
| 5.2–6.5mmol per litre | Increased |
| 6.5–7.5mmol per litre | Moderate |
| Greater than 7.5mmol per litre | High |

### High and low density lipoproteins

Cholesterol found in the blood is not all of the same type. Because it is a fatty substance, it is not soluble in water and has to be carried around in the blood stream by special proteins called lipoproteins. There are three types of lipoprotein, called high density lipoproteins (HDLs), low density lipoproteins (LDLs) and very low density lipoproteins (VLDLs). It is the HDLs and the LDLs that are of special importance in relation to heart disease. About 70 per cent of blood cholesterol is carried by LDLs, and high LDL levels are directly related to heart disease risk. Your LDL cholesterol level gives your doctor a better indication of your risk of heart disease than a total cholesterol level alone. The main role of LDLs is to supply cholesterol to body tissue. HDLs, on the other hand, appear to have a protective role, since they help to transport cholesterol away from the artery walls and return it to the liver for its conversion and excretion via bile salts.

**HDLs and LDLs and risk of heart disease**

Raised LDLs    →    Raised risk of heart disease

Low HDLs    →    Raised risk of heart disease

Raised HDLs    →    Low risk of heart disease

Before the menopause, women have higher HDL levels than men of the same age, which may partly explain the lower rate of heart disease in women before the onset of the menopause.

Remember: HDL = Healthy
    LDL = Less healthy

**Exercise and blood cholesterol levels**

All exercise, unless overdone, is good for the heart. Regular exercise reduces total blood cholesterol and increases the beneficial HDL cholesterol levels. It has the added bonus of being good for the figure and helps to combat stress. The best exercise for the heart is that which builds up stamina – the ability to keep going without running out of breath. To do this, you need regular exercise that is energetic enough to make you a little breathless and to raise your pulse rate.

Pick an activity that you enjoy, one that is convenient and one in which you will find satisfaction. There are many to choose from: brisk walking, swimming, cycling, jogging, exercising to dance music, tennis, and so on. Plan your program and make a commitment to it. Try to have some form of physical activity for 30 minutes, three times a week. It is easiest if you can build it into your normal routine. For example, use 30 minutes of your lunch hour to have your lunch and take a brisk walk for the remaining 30 minutes.

## *Weight and cholesterol levels*

Excess weight increases the workload of both heart and lungs. In an extensive American study on heart disease it was found that overweight people were twice as likely to suffer from heart disease as those who are not overweight. This is because obesity is closely associated with raised blood pressure, raised blood cholesterol and triglyceride levels, and decreased levels of HDL cholesterol. Overweight people also tend to exercise less.

It is therefore advisable, if you are overweight, to try to reduce it both by restricting your calorie intake (especially calories from fat and saturated fat) and by increasing the amount of exercise you take.

## Dietary cholesterol

Cholesterol in the diet is found in animal and sea foods only; rich sources include egg yolk, liver, kidney, fish roe and shellfish. Milk, cream, cheese and fatty meats, although not very rich sources, can contribute a significant amount when eaten in relatively large amounts.

It is important to understand that a low-cholesterol diet is not the same as a cholesterol-lowering diet. A diet that is low in cholesterol will have only a small, if any, effect of blood cholesterol levels.

A cholesterol-lowering diet is one in which the saturated fat is reduced and replaced with polyunsaturated and/or monounsaturated fat.

### How can you reduce blood cholesterol levels?

Dietary modification is the first and most important line of defence in lowering and controlling blood cholesterol levels. However, exercise and weight control also have a part to play.

Of the many dietary factors that have been studied on the relationship between diet, blood cholesterol and heart disease, dietary fat has proved to be the strongest and most consistent link.

### Saturated fats

Saturated fats are the villains of the piece when eaten in large quantities, since a high intake of saturated fat is associated with an increase in blood cholesterol levels. Saturated fat is mainly found in animal fats such as fat on meat, butter, hard animal cooking fats, e.g. dripping and lard, full fat milk, cheese and cream. Exceptions are coconut and palm oils, as well as solid vegetable shortenings and margarines that are made more saturated by a process called hydrogenation.

In general, the harder a fat is at room temperature, the more saturated it is. For instance, butter, which contains about 52 per cent saturated fat, is solid at room temperature, while corn or sunflower oil contain only 13 per cent saturates and are liquid at the same temperature.

## Unsaturated fats

**Monounsaturated fats:** monounsaturates were generally regarded as being fairly neutral in terms of health, but recent evidence suggests they have a beneficial effect on blood cholesterol levels. It has long been acknowledged that people living around the Mediterranean, who have a high intake of olive oil, have low rates of heart disease. However, their low rates of heart disease were attributed to a low intake of saturated fat rather than to their high intake of monounsaturated fats.

In recent years, since scientists have recognised the existence and importance of HDL cholesterol and LDL cholesterol in the prevention of heart disease, studies have shown that monounsaturates lower LDLs (the 'baddies') and raise HDLs. This contrasts with the polyunsaturated fats which lower both types of cholesterol. However, before rushing out to replace your high polyunsaturated fats with mononunsaturates, poly-unsaturates have a unique role to play in health because they are rich in 'essential' fatty acids which the body cannot make for itself.

Monounsaturates are commonly found in plant oils and foods. Rich sources include olive, rapeseed and groundnut oils as well as peanuts, olives and avocado pears. Almonds and hazelnuts are also high in monounsaturates. The most important fatty acid quantitatively in this group, is oleic acid.

**Polyunsaturated Fatty Acids (PUFAs):** oils and foods high in polyun-saturated fats include vegetable oils such as grapeseed, soya, corn and sunflower and margarines made from these oils or labelled 'high in polyunsaturates'. Oily fish, such as mackerel and herring, and nuts, such as walnuts, are also good sources. In the UK diet, linoleic acid is quantitatively the most important fatty acid in this group.

Polyunsaturates play a beneficial role in the prevention of heart disease in two ways:

- they lower blood cholesterol levels;
- they reduce the tendency of blood to clot.

Although there is a huge amount of evidence to show that polyunsatu-rated fats have a cholesterol-lowering effect, the way in which they do this is not fully understood. It is probably a combination of three things: they may help to reduce the production of cholesterol by the liver, to decrease the absorption of dietary cholesterol and to increase the excretion of cholesterol in the faeces. Of course, if they are replacing some of the saturated fat in the diet, that in itself will reduce blood cholesterol levels.

Polyunsaturated fatty acids inhibit the clumping together of blood platelets and so help to prevent blood clotting. Fish oil, which is rich in a polyunsaturated fatty acid called eicosapentanoic acid (EPA), is particularly effective in slowing down the clotting mechanism. This is why Eskimos, who eat so much fish and other marine food, have such a long bleeding time and low rate of heart disease. A number of studies have suggested that eating fish as little as twice a week protects against heart disease. This could be partly due to reducing the amount of saturated fat in the diet if meat meals are replaced with fish.

### Fibre in the diet

Studies suggest that high intakes of dietary fibre are associated with a reduced incidence of heart disease. The effect of fibre on blood cholesterol depends on the type of fibre consumed. Wheat fibre, for instance in bran or wholemeal bread, has only a small effect on blood cholesterol levels, but soluble fibre, such as pectin and guar, produces large reductions. Soluble fibre is found in oats, pulses such as peas and beans, fruit such as grapefruit and apples, and leafy vegetables like cabbage and spinach.

# —————— High blood pressure ——————

High blood pressure increases the risk of strokes and heart disease. It is more common in those who regularly drink large amounts of alcohol and those who are overweight. It is also more common in populations who have a relatively high salt intake. It is estimated that perhaps 10 per cent of the population are genetically susceptible to salt-related high blood pressure. In view of the fact that high blood pressure is often symptomless, should the whole population be advised to reduce their salt intake? The expert committee on Dietary Reference Values has cautioned against any trend towards increasing salt intakes, which it considers are already needlessly high.

For those who have been diagnosed as having high blood pressure, the best advice is as follows:

- If overweight, try to get down to the recommended weight for your height.
- Drink alcohol in moderation.
- Avoid salty foods; remember, 75 per cent of our salt comes from processed foods (see page 47).
- Avoid adding salt to food at table or in cooking.

## Prevention of heart disease – dietary advice

- Reduce overall fat intake.
- Reduce saturated (animal) fat.
- Increase fibre, especially soluble fibre.
- Eat plenty of vegetables and fruit.
- Use salt sparingly.
- Make sure you are the right weight for your height (see page 124).

# Food, nutrition and cancer

Normally, when the body needs to reproduce cells, such as during wound healing, this is done under some form of control that limits the number of cells produced to what is necessary. Cancer, however, is a disease or a family of diseases in which one or more cells in the body start to reproduce in an uncontrolled manner.

Cancer is the second leading cause of death in the UK, accounting for 23 per cent of all deaths, with lung, breast and colon cancers being the most common sites. It claims over 160,000 lives each year in the UK, yet we can all help ourselves to avoid cancer by being aware of risk factors.

It is estimated that 80 per cent of cancers are related to environmental factors and are, therefore, potentially preventable. The strong environmental influence is demonstrated by the change in incidence of cancer in migrant populations such as, for example, has occurred in Japanese migrants to the United States – mortality from breast and colon cancers is low in Japan and mortality from stomach cancer is high; in the United States the reverse is true. Within two or three generations, the pattern changed in the immigrant Japanese to that of the Americans. Similar patterns have been seen in Puerto Ricans migrating to the USA.

The EC has developed an 'awareness' programme, with a target of reducing deaths from cancer in Europe by 15 per cent by the year 2000. They have pinpointed smoking, poor diet and overexposure to ultraviolet light as major causes of cancer. We, as individuals, can control each of these factors.

The famous epidemiologist, Sir Richard Doll, has suggested that possibly 35 per cent of all types of cancer may be linked to diet, 30 per cent to tobacco, 3 per cent to alcohol, 1 per cent to food additives and 1 per cent to food contamination and industrial pollution.

## Diet

Although it is difficult to find hard proof to link cancer with poor diet, some experts believe about 30–40 per cent of cancers in men and up to 60 per cent of cancers in women are linked to what we eat. The relationship between specific dietary components and cancer is much less well established than between diet and heart disease. However, the overall impact of diet on cancer rates around the world appears to be important. The cancers most commonly associated with dietary factors are cancers of the mouth, pharynx (behind nose and mouth), larynx (voice box), gullet, stomach, large bowel, liver, pancreas, breast and prostate. The table below shows, for example, that the higher the intake of fruit and vegetables, the lower the risk of developing various cancers.

| | fat | fibre | alcohol | fruit and vegetables | smoked/ pickled/ salted foods |
|---|---|---|---|---|---|
| Mouth | | | positive | negative | |
| Gullet | | | positive | negative | positive |
| Stomach | | | | negative | positive |
| Liver | | | positive | | |
| Colon/ rectum | positive | negative | positive | negative | |
| Prostate | positive | | | negative | |
| Lung | | | | negative | |
| Breast | positive | | | | |

Association between dietary components and cancer
Adapted from *Diet, nutrition and the prevention of chronic diseases*, (WHO, 1990)

## Fat

The US National Research Committee on Diet, Nutrition and Cancer concluded that, of all the dietary components it studied, the strongest evidence of a causal relationship between diet and cancer was with total fat intake. There is consistent evidence that increasing the intake of fat increases the incidence of cancer at certain sites, particularly the breast and colon, and conversely, that the risk is lower with lower fat intakes. Cancer of the prostate and ovarian cancers have also been associated with a high intake of fat.

In studies comparing different populations, the incidence of cancer correlates more with total fat rather than with any one type of dietary fat. However, experiments with animals suggest that vegetable oils containing omega-6 polyunsaturated fatty acids (see pages 9–14) promote cancer more effectively than saturated fat, whereas fish oils containing omega-3 fatty acids tend to inhibit tumour growth.

## Cholesterol in the blood

Several studies have linked very low blood cholesterol levels with increased risk of developing cancer. However, it has also been suggested that very low blood cholesterol levels may be an early indicator of the beginning of cancer rather than a cause of cancer.

In contrast, there is also some evidence that high blood cholesterol levels are associated with increased risk of cancer. This could, however, be because high cholesterol levels are associated with excessive fat consumption.

## Vitamins

Deficiencies of some vitamins seem to enhance tumour growth; vitamins C, E, A and the precursor of vitamin A, beta carotene, are all antioxidants which help to prevent body cells from being broken down and destroyed. A number of studies have suggested that a high consumption of these vitamins can help prevent degenerative diseases such as cancer.

**Vitamin A** deficiency in animals enhances their susceptibility to the induction of some tumours and retards or inhibits tumour development. The reasons for this are not understood, but the positive results of limited clinical trials suggest that vitamin A may have a beneficial effect when combined with chemotherapy.

**Vitamin E** has been shown to inhibit pre-cancerous cells from developing into tumours in animals. However, a lot more research is needed before any firm conclusions can be drawn.

**Vitamin C** blood levels have been found to be low in patients suffering from cancer. Indirect evidence on the association between cancer and vitamin C has come from studies showing that a high consumption of fruit and vegetables that contain a lot of vitamin C is linked with a lower risk of some forms of cancer.

## Fibre

Diets high in fibre have been associated with a reduced incidence of bowel cancer. This has stemmed from observations that communities who have a diet high in fibre have a lower incidence of bowel cancer than communities such as ours, who consume a relatively low amount of fibre. Of course, no single component of the diet can change without other components changing as well, and fibre intake affects all sorts of other things like meat, fat and vitamin intakes. It is not clear whether it is the fibre *per se* that has a protective role or whether it could be that foods containing fibre, such as fruit and cereals, generally contain other dietary elements, such as vitamins, which could have a protective role against cancer.

## Alcohol

Drinking alcohol is related to cancers of the upper part of the digestive tract: the mouth, pharynx, oesophagus and larynx. The risk of cancer seems to be increased in heavy drinkers who also smoke. Alcohol could play a role either directly as a cell toxin or as a vehicle for some non-alcoholic components (conveners) in alcoholic beverages, or it may be causal indirectly by depressing the immune response.

Dietary deficiencies combined with alcohol abuse may also increase the incidence of some cancers; in particular, associations have been found between alcohol consumption, low levels of the antioxidant vitamins A and E and tumour growth. Vitamin B6 plays an important role in the production of antibodies and is also thought to retard tumour development.

# *Pickles*

A high consumption of pickled vegetables has been linked to cancer of the gullet. These foods contain high concentrations of N-nitroso compounds

– nitrogen containing chemicals – which appear to be responsible for the increase in risk.

## Nitrates and nitrites

Nitrates are used widely in fertilisers and are found in small amounts in food, particularly vegetables. Nitrites are also used as a preservative (E250) in curing meat. Nitrate itself is not considered harmful but it can be broken down in the body to nitrite which can, under certain conditions, form nitrosamines. These nitrosamines cause stomach cancer in animals. However, no relationship has been found in humans between stomach cancer and consumption of vegetables, which is the main source of nitrate in the diet; in fact, the opposite is true – the consumption of vegetables is associated with a lower risk of stomach cancer. This may be because vegetables contain vitamin C, which is known to inhibit nitrosamine formation.

## Conclusion

It is not possible, on the basis of current knowledge, to quantify the contribution of diet to different cancers. However, the evidence is sufficiently strong to suggest that a diet low in fat, alcohol, salted, pickled and smoked foods and high in plant foods, especially those high in carotene and vitamin C, is consistent with a low risk of many cancers.

## Cancer prevention – summary of advice

- Give up smoking.
- Eat plenty of fresh fruit and vegetables to increase your intake of vitamin C and beta-carotene (vitamin A).
- Eat plenty of wholegrain cereal foods to increase your fibre intake.
- Limit your intake of fatty foods.
- Moderate your alcohol intake.
- Minimise consumption of foods preserved by pickling, salt-curing and smoking.
- Avoid over-exposure to direct sunlight.

# — Nutrition and the immune system —

The body's immune system is on constant alert to recognise foreign invasion and to act against infective agents. The immune system recognises not just bacteria and viruses but also healthy tissues from another human being as 'foreign', which is why organ transplants are sometimes rejected.

The importance of the relationship between the immune system and nutrition is increasingly recognised. It is also now generally acknowledged that the relationship is important not only in countries where there is severe malnutrition with a high incidence of infectious diseases, but also in populations with relatively mild forms of malnourishment or even single nutrient deficiency. A wide variety of nutrients, essential for survival and for good health, have been shown to have an impact on immune function. The interaction of proteins, vitamins and minerals, all of which must originate from the diet, is required for the formation of immunoglobulins and enzymes, which play an important role in the immune system.

The influence of nutrient intake on immune function is only one aspect: most forms of disease, whether acute or chronic, result in increased requirements of many nutrients. Vitamins can be lost from the body as a result of stresses ranging from infections, such as coughs and colds, to anxiety states, emotional strain or continuous pain. Any increase in metabolism means an increase in the need for the B vitamins, particularly B1, B2 and B3 (thiamin, riboflavin and niacin).

The first line of defence is the actual barrier to infective agents – the skin and mucous membranes (lining the throat, respiratory tract, etc.). These tissues need vitamin A to keep them in good order so that they can function properly. That is why vitamin A is often referred to as the 'anti-infective' vitamin.

The body has two types of defence after this. One is secretory, that is in the fluids, such as blood, tears and saliva, which produce antibodies in response to invading toxins. The other type of defence is cellular, where cells are produced at local sites of infection to destroy the invading bacteria.

Many vitamins are involved in these defence systems. Vitamins A, B6 and folic acid are required for the production of antibodies. Vitamins A, B6, B12, C and folic acid are all involved in cellular defence. A shortage of any one of these vitamins will, therefore, impair the body's defences.

People often find they lose their appetite during times of illness. A vicious circle can occur, where lack of food means lack of essential nutrients to help combat the infection and so leads to further reduce a person's ability to return to good health. The nutrients most likely to suffer are those which are not stored in appreciable amounts by the body – the water-soluble B vitamins and vitamin C.

Although some nutrients may be of particular relevance to the immune system, it is important to consider the level of all nutrients in the diet, since there are complex interactions between many of them; for instance, although a person's iron intake may appear to be sufficient, without adequate vitamin C iron absorption will be less efficient. Likewise, an overdose of a supplement of an individual mineral, such as zinc, will compete and interfere with the absorption of other important minerals such as calcium.

Consumption of highly refined and heavily processed foods in which trace elements and vitamin contents can be reduced substantially can contribute to low nutrient status in Western society. It is, therefore, important to ensure a diet which contains lots of fresh, unprocessed, unrefined foods, such as fruit, vegetables and wholegrain cereals, which will provide both fibre and essential nutrients to maximise your chances of a fit and healthy body, ready to combat illnesses for you and all the family.

# Polyunsaturated fat and inflammatory diseases

Diets rich in eicosapentanoic acid (EPA), an omega-3 fatty acid which is found in fish oil, reduce inflammatory reactions. Similar changes occur with the omega-6 fatty acid gamma-linolenic acid (GLA), found in borage oil and evening primrose oil. Almost all chronic diseases with an immunological component, including multiple sclerosis, bronchial asthma, rheumatoid arthritis and the inflammatory skin diseases eczema and psoriasis, have been the subject of scientific studies. The results so far have been disappointing for multiple sclerosis supplemented with EPA. However, the results using the parent omega-6 fatty acid, linoleic acid found in sunflower and other common culinary oils (see the graph on page 64), have been more encouraging in terms of benefit in relapse rates and rate of progression of the disease. There was no clinical improvement for asthma sufferers. The results for rheumatoid arthritis and EPA have been more consistent in reducing the severity by reducing morning stiffness and joint swelling. Modest improvements were found in inflammatory skin disorders.

Chronic inflammatory diseases, by definition, run over a long period of time and are marked by unpredictable remissions and relapses. It is therefore difficult to recommend that such oil supplements should be given routinely in inflammatory disorders. These are still early days in terms of research, and no doubt much more will be understood about the relationship between polyunsaturated fatty acids and the immune system in the years to come.

# ——— Nutrition, HIV and AIDS ———

Human Immunodeficiency Virus (HIV) attacks the immune system and, under certain conditions, the disease may progress to Acquired Immune Deficiency Syndrome (AIDS). This devastating disease renders its victims defenceless against infection. Currently AIDS has no cure. Treatments focus on slowing down the course of the disease and controlling the symptoms. The severe wasting associated with AIDS is multifactorial. Inadequate food intake is often brought on by depression over the diagnosis, even before symptoms of the disease appear. Excessive nutrient losses due to malabsorption and diarrhoea, nutrient-drug interactions, appetite suppression due to drugs and repeated infections all contribute to accelerating weight loss.

A positive result for HIV infection should alert the individual and health care workers to the need for aggressive nutrition intervention. It is important for sufferers to maintain a good diet because vitamin and mineral deficiencies have an adverse effect on immune function, and malnutrition may contribute to the progression of the disease. A nutritionally balanced diet from early in the course of the disease is needed to help prevent weight loss and to maximise the body's immune function. If the sufferer is not eating well, it is a good idea to take a good vitamin/mineral supplement, but there is no good evidence that mega-doses of particular vitamins or other dietary supplements, such as geranium, can boost the immune response. Because AIDS sufferers are at increased risk of infection, they are best advised to avoid eating foods like raw eggs and soft rinded cheeses (see pages 159–161).

# Nutrition-related problems in adulthood

## *Premenstrual tension and diet*

Premenstrual tension (PMT) is a term used to cover a range of symptoms that can occur during the second half of the monthly cycle when a fall in hormone levels occurs. It is a problem that affects many women, and the symptoms may be physical or psychological. Physical symptoms vary from person to person, but the most common include abdominal swelling due to water retention, headaches, breast tenderness and backache. The psychological symptoms include marked mood swings, depression, lack of concentration, tension and irritability. All in all, PMT can cause a lot of misery and disruption both to family and working life.

While it must be emphasised that no PMT treatment helps every PMT sufferer, many women have been relieved of several of the symptoms by dietary intervention, most notably by use of vitamin B6 (pyridoxine) and evening primrose oil.

### Vitamin B6 and PMT

There is no evidence that women who suffer from PMT have lower vitamin B6 levels than others and, in general, few of the properly conducted studies report much benefit from doses of vitamin B6 between 50mg and 200mg per day. Yet despite this lack of scientific evidence, vitamin B6 is widely prescribed and self-prescribed for the treatment of PMT.

Vitamin B6 has been found to help some women who suffer from depression while on oral contraceptives, which are known to reduce vitamin B6 blood levels. This led to studies on the use of vitamin B6 in the treatment of PMT. The evidence remains uncertain: some women have reported improvements with supplementation, particularly for pre-menstrual headache, bloating, depression and irritability. It is always unsatisfactory to be presented with information that is not clearcut, but the best advice for PMT sufferers is probably to try supplementation for about three menstrual cycles and document for themselves any changes they feel supplementation makes.

It is important not to take very large doses – no more than 200mg a day. High doses of vitamin B6 (in excess of 500mg per day) have been shown to cause nerve damage and even more modest doses cannot be regarded as being without hazard.

**Evening primrose oil and PMT**

An alternative nutritional approach to PMT has been supplementation with evening primrose oil, which has a high concentration of the poly-unsaturated fatty acid gamma-linolenic acid, which is used by the body to make regulatory substances. Studies in both England and Sweden have reported a reduction in PMT symptoms in some but not all sufferers. The usual dose is two or three capsules of evening primrose oil twice daily after food.

The mechanism by which gamma-linolenic acid is effective in PMT is not known, but it has been suggested that PMT may be observed in women with a minor abnormality in converting the parent omega-6 fatty acid (see pages 9–14) to gamma-linolenic acid, which helps to regulate hormone levels. Some sufferers of PMT have found a combination of evening primrose oil and vitamin B6 (50–75mg per day) more helpful than when taken separately.

Anyone suffering from PMT should ensure they have plenty of fresh fruit, vegetables and wholegrain cereals and bread, which will help to ensure they have a good supply of B vitamins and vitamin C, as well as minerals such as magnesium.

## Osteoporosis

From about the age of 35, bones gradually start to lose more calcium than they take up. This leads to a slow loss of bone density and, like greying of hair, is a normal consequence of ageing. The overall size of the bone remains the same but the bones become less dense, more fragile and more liable to fracture. Hence the Greek word 'osteoporosis', *osteo* meaning bone. This loss of bone accelerates in women after the meno-pause, increasing their susceptibility to fractures. About one in four women over the age of 60 will have an osteoporosis-related fracture, compared to one in 40 men.

Although you probably think of your bones as solid objects of fixed composition, in fact calcium is constantly moving in and out of them. This 're-modelling' of bone varies with age. In a young child whose bones are growing quickly, the skeleton can be entirely replaced in one to two years, while in an adult, complete renewal will take about seven to ten years providing, of course, the amount of calcium in the diet is sufficient to meet requirements. Bones stop growing in length in the late teens but will continue to increase in density and strength well into the twenties when they reach their peak strength.

## Osteoporosis – preventable?

Osteoporosis, like other degenerative changes related to age, cannot be prevented, but there are three separate ways which may be useful in slowing down its rate of progress: hormone replacement therapy (HRT), plenty of exercise and a good diet with an adequate intake of calcium.

Hormone replacement therapy replaces oestrogen, which reduces the rate at which bone calcium is lost. The prolonged use of oestrogen after the menopause carries some of its own dangers as well as benefits and is therefore not always considered to be the ideal preventive measure. Physical exercise also helps to prevent loss of bone density.

## Diet

Many women have been led to believe that dosing themselves with large amounts of calcium supplements or drinking calcium fortified milks will help strengthen their bones. This is not, however, usually recommended because it can interfere with absorption of other minerals.

The first step in prevention begins in childhood: a good diet with plenty of calcium and lots of exercise all help to build strong bones. A high calcium intake during childhood and adolescence, before peak bone mass occurs, seems to be the most effective means of ensuring good bone density in later life. That said, because there is a constant turnover of calcium in bones, it is important to have an adequate intake of calcium throughout life.

| Group | | Age (years) | Calcium per day (mg) |
|---|---|---|---|
| Children | | 1–3 | 350 |
| | | 4–6 | 450 |
| | | 7–10 | 550 |
| Adolescent | girls | 11–18 | 800 |
| | boys | 11–18 | 1,000 |
| Adult | women | 19+ | 700 |
| | men | 19+ | 700 |
| Pregnant women | | | no increment |
| Breast-feeding women | | | +550 |

Requirements for calcium per day
Crown copyright. Reproduced with the permission of the Controller of HMSO.

| Food | Amount (average portion) | Calcium (mg) |
|---|---|---|
| Yoghurt | 150g tub | 225 |
| Sardines (120g tin, drained) | 100g | 550 |
| Milk, whole | 0.5 pint | 325 |
| Milk, skimmed | 0.5 pint | 340 |
| Figs, dried | 5 (100g) | 280 |
| Salmon, tinned (inc. bones) | 100g | 240 |
| Cheese, Edam | 1oz/28g | 218 |
| Cheese, Cheddar | 1oz/28g | 204 |
| Spinach, boiled | 3.5oz/100g | 160 |
| Bread, white | 3 medium slices | 100 |
| Spring greens, boiled | 3.5oz/100g | 86 |
| Orange | 1 medium | 60 |

Calcium-rich foods
Data/information from *The Composition of Foods*, 5th ed. (1991) is reproduced with the permission of the Royal Society of Chemistry and the Controller of HMSO.

# Gout

Gout is a form of arthritis characterised by increased quantities of uric acid in the blood. Uric acid is an end product of purine metabolism, formed in the breakdown of protein and arising from normal wear and tear of body tissues and cell turnover. The uric acid crystallises out in the small joints, typically in the big toe, causing very acute pain. It usually occurs in middle age and is much more common in men, particularly those who are overweight and those who regularly drink alcohol. Alcohol is thought to inhibit the excretion of uric acid, and an acute attack can often be precipitated by over-indulgence in alcohol.

## Treatment

Gout is usually treated quite successfully with a drug that inhibits uric acid production, such as allopurinol, or with a urate-eliminating drug which decreases the uric acid blood level by increasing the amount eliminated by the kidneys. Part of the reason for the success of drugs over dietary restrictions is that dietary sources of uric acid contribute at most 50 per cent of the uric acid found in blood; the rest is formed within the body and seems to bear very little relationship to the amount of exogenous or dietary purine. Nevertheless, gout is generally a disease of plenty, and during times of hardship and deprivation, as happened during the two World Wars, gout rarely occurred.

## Diet

Because of the efficiency of modern drug treatment, drugs have largely replaced the need for rigid dietary restrictions. However, during acute phases in particular, restriction of purine-rich foods is recommended so as not to add to the existing high uric acid load. These include organ meats, such as liver, kidney and sweetbreads, as well as yeast, meat extracts and oily fish including sardines, mackerel and herring, shellfish and fish roes.

# 7

## VEGETARIANS AND VEGANS

───────────── **Vegetarianism** ─────────────

In recent years, ecological, humane and health factors have attracted many people to vegetarianism. It is argued, for instance, that it is wasteful of the earth's limited resources to feed plants to animals and then eat the animals – an acre of land can produce ten times as much vegetable protein as it can from meat protein, if used for grazing cattle.

There are several levels of vegetarianism, all of which exclude different animal foods from their diet. All vegetarians exclude meat and fish. A lacto-vegetarian includes milk and milk products; an ova-vegetarian includes eggs, but a vegan, or strict vegetarian, eats no food of animal origin at all. Their diet consists entirely of vegetables, vegetable oils, cereals and fruit.

Fruitarianism is an extreme form of veganism, which excludes not just foods of animal origin but also pulses and cereals. A fruitarian diet consists mainly of raw and dried fruit, nuts, honey and olive oil. It is not possible for such a diet to meet nutritional requirements.

### Do vegetarian diets provide adequate nutrition?

Nutritional deficiencies can occur, particularly when an individual simply stops eating animal products without considering what they will replace those foods with. It is therefore important that some general principles are understood.

## Calories

Vegetarian diets can readily meet energy (calorie) intakes, providing enough food is eaten.

## Protein

Milk, milk products and eggs are all rich sources of protein for the lacto-ova-vegetarians. Pulses, nuts and seeds all contain protein, as do many plant foods such as bread and other cereal products. However, for the vegan, in order to obtain an adequate supply of all the amino acids which make up protein and which have specific essential functions, it is necessary to eat a mixture of plant proteins. So, as long as a variety of plant proteins is eaten, i.e. from cereal grains, pulses, nuts and seeds, the amino acids they contain will complement each other. In this way, any deficits in one plant protein will be compensated for by the amino acids in another.

## Vitamins

The fat-soluble vitamins A (in the form of beta-carotene) and E are found naturally in plant foods, and our main source of vitamin D is from the action of sunlight on our skin.

The water-soluble vitamin C and the B vitamins are all present in plant foods, with the exception of vitamin B12. Strict vegetarians or vegans are therefore at risk of developing deficiency. In most vegans, their B12 blood levels are often reduced, and they may experience a sore mouth and tongue, but anaemia is unusual. It is not understood how vegans do obtain vitamin B12; it is thought there may be traces in micro-organisms and mould which contaminate their food.

## Minerals

Concern has been voiced about both iron and zinc intakes in vegetarian diets. This is because the best sources of these two nutrients are meat and meat products. Vegans, who exclude milk and milk products, are also at risk of having a low calcium intake. About 20 per cent of the iron in our diet comes from meat, which is particularly well absorbed in comparison to non-meat iron sources, e.g. cereals, green vegetables, pulses and eggs. However, the absorption of iron is enhanced by vitamin C, which is often high in vegetarian diets. This, together with a suggestion that vegetarians may adapt to lower intakes by increased absorption, may explain why most studies have not found iron deficiency to be a problem for most vegetarian/vegans. Studies on zinc status have been conflicting, but there is no strong evidence as yet to suggest that vegetarians and vegans are seriously at risk of zinc deficiency. As might be expected, lacto-vegetarians have relatively high intakes of calcium. Vegans, on the other hand, have substantially lower intakes of calcium than vegetarians, although there have been no reports of calcium deficiency in adult vegans. It may be that vegans can conserve calcium more efficiently or, as is known, calcium absorption becomes more efficient when calcium intakes fall and at times of increased need, as in pregnancy.

## Children on vegetarian/vegan diets

Lacto-ova-vegetarian diets can support growth, even in very young children, as can carefully planned vegan diets. However, malnutrition can and does arise in children, particularly when parents do not have sufficient information to avoid making mistakes in food choice. One of the main problems for young children is that these diets are bulky in relation to their energy content, and it is difficult to fulfil energy requirements for sustained growth. Nutrients likely to be low in a vegan diet and which children in particular may benefit from supplementing are calcium, iron, vitamin B2 (found in milk), vitamin B12 and vitamin D. Like vegan children, lacto-ovo-vegetarian children have been found to be slightly smaller in stature and lighter than non-vegetarian children, but the studies have been limited and more research is needed.

## Are vegetarians healthier?

There have been many studies comparing disease incidence in vegetarians and meat eaters, including heart disease, obesity, blood pressure and cancer. Vegetarians have a much lower rate of heart disease: vegetarians generally have diets which are lower in fat and saturated fat and higher in fibre, which may in part explain this difference. However, many other aspects of lifestyle, such as smoking, may vary between meat eaters and vegetarians, so it is difficult to attribute this difference solely to diet. They also tend to have slightly lower blood pressure levels. Vegetarians are less likely to be overweight than non-vegetarians. Their higher fibre intake may contribute to this, but it could also be that they are less likely to eat less healthy, high energy dense foods such as high-sugar foods or alcohol. Some types of cancer are also less frequently seen in vegetarians; again, while this could be partly attributed to lower fat, higher fibre intakes, it could also be due to the healthier lifestyles of many vegetarians.

## Conclusion

There are good and bad vegetarian-type diets, but when properly planned, they may overall have positive health benefits. It is especially important to ensure young children and pregnant and breast-feeding women have an adequate supply of energy and essential nutrients.

## *Checklist*

- **Energy:** for those with small appetites and for children, it is necessary to include energy-dense foods, including nuts, nut butters, oil, margarine, milk or milk substitutes, cheese and/or yoghurts.
- **Protein:** it is important to have a mixture of sources of vegetable proteins, i.e. nuts, seeds, pulses, cereals including bread, milk substitutes or milk, cheese and eggs if eaten.
- **Vitamins**
  (a) Vitamin B12 – try to have B12 fortified foods, such as yeast extracts like Barmene; some soya milks (e.g. Plamil) and breakfast cereals which are also fortified, e.g. Grapenuts (check labels). If these are not eaten, take a vitamin B12 supplement.
  (b) Vitamin D – exposure to sunlight is important; fortified breakfast cereals, milk and eggs are also good sources.
  (c) Vitamin B2 – milk and eggs if eaten, green leafy vegetables, wholegrain cereals and bread, fortified breakfast cereals.
- **Minerals**
  (a) Iron – pulses, wholegrain cereals and bread, dried fruit, wheatgerm, nuts and green vegetables are all good sources of iron. Eggs contain iron, but an absorption-inhibiting factor in eggs makes them a poor source.
  (b) Calcium – milk and cheese if eaten, fortified milk substitutes, sesame seeds, nuts, cereals and bread, green vegetables such as broccoli and hard water.

# 8

# NUTRITION AND SPORT

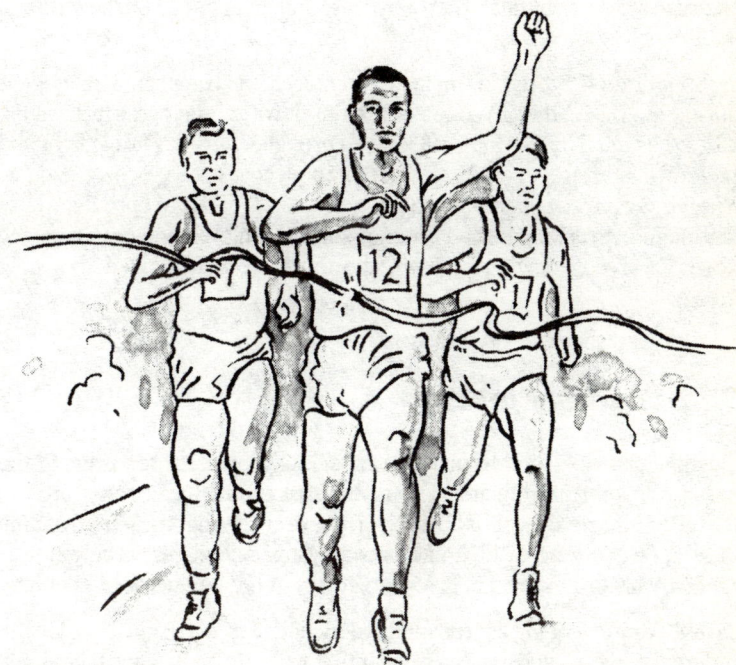

Like many other areas of nutrition, there are some confusing and often misinformed messages about the potential benefits of megavitamins, protein supplements, royal jelly, kelp, wheat germ, honey, ginseng and other 'health' preparations. Few of the theories attached to these claims have any scientific backing to support them. Developing and maintaining physical fitness is not about pumping vitamins or other supplements into your body; there is no magical approach to putting 'a tiger in your tank' or building a body beautiful. That said, much research is now going on into the role of nutrition and diet management in improving physical performance, and no doubt a lot more will be understood about diet and physical activity in the next decade.

Energy is, of course, of primary importance when carrying out any physical activity. Requirements depend on a number of factors: besides sex, age and body size, type of exercise, intensity, duration and frequency of activity all need to be taken into consideration. Energy comes principally from carbohydrate, fat and protein. In the normal, well-fed individual, protein does not contribute very much to energy production, since it is being used for tissue maintenance, growth and other purposes. The relative contribution of carbohydrate and fat depends on the duration and intensity of exercise.

Carbohydrate is stored in the liver and muscles in the form of glycogen. During exercise, this glycogen is broken down to glucose which, along with fat, is used by working muscles to provide energy. During light and moderate exercise, the muscles use both glycogen, as glucose, and fat. When this exercise increases in intensity, e.g. repeated sprinting, or is continued over a long period of time, such as long-distance running, the stores of glycogen will run down and more fat will be used to supply energy.

## Carbohydrate loading

This is a practice used to increase muscle glycogen stores prior to the endurance sporting events. The aim is to increase glycogen stores to above their normal level. It is based on the premise that the length of time an athlete can sustain high-intensity physical activity is largely determined by his or her level of glycogen stores at the beginning of exercise.

Carbohydrate loading is recommended only for occasional prolonged endurance events and not as a regular dietary pattern. The most common procedure is to consume a high-carbohydrate diet (70 per cent of energy) in the form of starchy foods, such as pasta, bread, rice and potatoes, for three or four days before the event; during this time the athlete should undertake only light training. On the day of the event, the athlete should have a high-carbohydrate meal no later than three to four hours before the start of the event.

# Fluid balance

Inadequate hydration is a major cause of poor performance during physical activity, especially during hot weather. Fluid loss can be as much as two litres per hour during two or three hours of exercise. The Food and Nutrition Board suggests that impaired performance occurs with a 3 per cent body weight loss, heat exhaustion with a 5 per cent loss and collapse with a 10 per cent loss. These losses are unlikely to occur with short intense bouts of exercise but have been observed in long-distance events such as marathons and cycling. Thirst is not an adequate indication of fluid requirement, and so athletes need to discipline themselves to take appropriate fluid replacement. A good rule of thumb is to start with three or more glasses of liquid about three hours before the event, take another two glasses about an hour and a half before and continue to take at least two glasses every hour during the event. With prolonged exercise, it is not possible to replenish fluid loss during performance due to the large amounts that would be required, so it is also necessary to continue rehydration after physical activity. Water is generally considered to be the best choice for fluid replacement. However, during prolonged exercise, a weak glucose solution will help 'spare' muscle glycogen and delay fatigue. It is important that the solution should be weak (hypotonic), i.e. 2–2.5g per 100ml of water, as more concentrated solutions slow down absorption. Aerated drinks should be avoided before and during exercise.

# Vitamins and minerals

Despite the widespread use of vitamins and minerals among athletes, there is no scientific evidence that either will improve the performance of someone who is already well nourished. Of course, correction of deficiencies due to improper diet will improve performance, but prevention of such deficiencies is best tackled by means of a balanced and varied diet.

The only vitamins in which there may be an increase in requirements are those involved in the breakdown of energy-yielding nutrients. These include vitamins B1 (thiamin), B2 (riboflavin) and B3 (niacin). However, for the most part, it can be expected that the requirements of these will be met by any increase in food consumption.

Anaemia in athletes can impair physical performance, because the iron in red blood cells plays a role in the transport of oxygen from the lungs to the tissues, and in respiration. An adequate intake of iron is, therefore, of special importance for those who are involved in endurance sports, which put a high demand on oxygen uptake. Iron supplements will help the performance of those who are iron deficient, as measured by biochemical markers of iron status, but are of no benefit to those with a satisfactory iron status.

# 9
# FOOD SAFETY

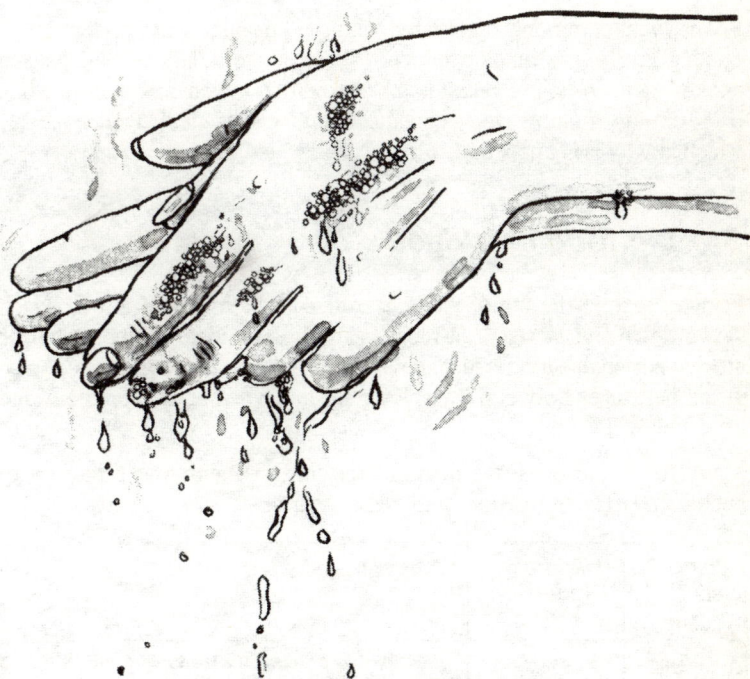

## Food hygiene

Although some food-borne infections, such as cholera, typhoid fever and brucellosis, are now rare diseases, some infections, such as salmonellosis and campylobacter enteritis, are on the increase and remain an major public health problem. The most common form of food poisoning in the home is caused by contamination of food with the bacteria salmonella.

Food spoilage is caused by a number of things, including the environment (e.g. air, light, warmth), micro-organisms (e.g. bacteria, moulds) and enzymes which stimulate chemical changes. Shelf life is also influenced by the composition of the food itself: foods high in saturated fat, such as fat in meat, will stay fresh longer than polyunsaturated fats as found, for instance, in fish.

Some people are more prone to food poisoning than others, in particular babies, elderly people, pregnant women and people who are ill and have a low resistance to infection. These groups need to be extra vigilant about avoiding the risk of food poisoning.

Foods most commonly associated with food poisoning are undercooked poultry and eggs, meat products, shellfish, soft-rinded cheeses and cooked rice. Food poisoning is more common in warm weather, when bacteria can multiply very quickly. Salmonella is destroyed by heat, which is why it is important to cook poultry and eggs thoroughly.

## Storing food in fridges

Fridges extend the life of foods by reducing their temperature, which slows down the increase of most bacteria. The ideal temperature for storing perishable food is just above freezing point. Most fridges operate at temperatures between 1 and 7°C and should be set to keep the fridge at or below 5°C.

Many fridges also have a deep-freeze compartment; the capability of such compartments varies from one to four stars.

| Star rating | Approx. temperature setting | Capability |
| --- | --- | --- |
| * star | −6°C | Already frozen food for up to one week. |
| ** stars | −12°C | Already frozen food for up to one month. |
| *** stars | −18°C | Already frozen food for up to three months. |
| **** stars | −18°C | Proper freezer compartments which can freeze unfrozen food and keep it for up to three months. |

To avoid cross-contamination, foods such as raw meat or defrosting foods should be stored in covered dishes or boxes which can catch drips. It is best to keep these foods underneath any cooked foods, which should also be covered to avoid air-borne contamination. Make sure foods do not drip on to salads and vegetables in the vegetable drawer.

## Summary – to avoid the risk of food poisoning

- Wash your hands before handling food.
- Defrost food thoroughly before cooking.
- Store raw food separately from cooked food.
- Avoid food from sources where standards of hygiene are questionable.
- Don't eat food which has passed its 'use-by' date.
- Don't eat raw eggs.
- Keep your fridge at the correct temperature (below 5°C).
- Take chilled and frozen foods home as quickly as possible.
- Keep pets away from food and worktops.
- Reheat cooked foods thoroughly.
- Use separate chopping boards and knives for raw meat and other foods.

# Food additives

Food additives are substances which are deliberately added to processed foods to prevent spoilage, to improve quality in terms of taste, texture, colour or nutritional value and to aid processing. For example, calcium propionate (E282) may be added to bread to prevent mould growth, vitamin B1 to breakfast cereals to improve nutritional content, or carrageen, a seaweed (E407), may be added to ice-cream as an emulsifier.

Additives are now listed with the ingredients of packaged foods. Although they have a generic name, such as ascorbic acid, they also have a European Community number, the 'E' number. All E numbers have been tested and passed for safety by the EC. Numbers without an E are permitted in the UK, but not passed by all EC countries. These are not declared as such on labels but by their name.

So many scare stories appeared in the press in the 1980s that many consumers started to take E numbers as a health warning rather than a guarantee of their safety, as intended by the EC. This has prompted food manufacturers to revert to listing many additives by their name so as not to prejudice the consumer.

Food additives, for many people, are conceived as being something artificial. In fact, this is a misconception, as many additives are substances that occur in nature, for example, lecithin and ascorbic acid, which is vitamin C. Additives are not always the products of twentieth-century technology. Our ancestors used salt to preserve meats and fish, preserved fruit in sugar and vegetables, such as onions, in vinegar. Artificial additives are those which have been synthesised or are a natural product that has been chemically modified. Only artificial additives are given E numbers, so natural substances, such as herbs, salt and sugar, do not have E numbers.

## Are additives safe?

Food additives have an emotive ring to them, but without additives, the variety of food available would be severely curtailed, since much food processing could not take place. All additives have to be safe and effective, as well as necessary, before their use is permitted. The main objections to food additives are that:

- a small number of individuals show adverse reactions to certain additives such as tartrazine (E102) and benzoic acid (E210);
- they allow food manufacturers to sell bulking agents, such as air and water, at inflated prices;
- they can be used to disguise poor quality foods such as fatty meat in sausages.

A government-appointed committee of experts judges whether additives should be permitted. Food activists frequently charge that such committees have too high a proportion of experts from within the food industry. Since most people working with food additives might be expected to be allied to food manufacturing, this is perhaps not surprising or even unreasonable and, as in many professional situations, professional reputations are very important to the individual, so abuse of their position is unlikely.

Food activists have been criticised by the food scientists as using unconfirmed reports to support their theories and using as evidence side effects in situations where unrealistically high levels of an additive were consumed.

## Additives by category

The main groups of additives are preservatives, colourings, emulsifiers, stabilisers and flavourings.

### Preservatives

These form the most important class of food additives because they help to prevent food spoilage. They help to ensure all-year-round supplies of palatable, safe food. There are two main types of preservatives: anti-microbial agents (E numbers from E200 to E299) and antioxidants (E300 to E322).

Antimicrobial agents help to prevent growth of moulds, yeasts and bacteria, such as salmonella and clostridium botulinum, which can make food inedible and sometimes poisonous.

Antioxidants stop oils, fats and fat-soluble vitamins in food from being destroyed and going rancid. They also help to stop the enzyme action that causes fruit, such as apples, and vegetables, such as potatoes, to turn brown when they are sliced.

In an attempt to achieve public approval, some food producers are removing preservatives from their products. There are, however, some disadvantages in that the consumer ends up with a product that stays safe and palatable for a shorter period of time.

### Colourings

These additives are put in food mainly to make them look more appetising and compensate for colour loss in processing. Many consumers see these as least necessary, and manufacturers have been criticised for covering up for over-processing. Unfortunately, we have been condi-tioned to expect tinned peas to be green and strawberry jam to be red, and the public are unlikely to buy visually unappetising foods. Some progress has been made in that some manufacturers now colour orange squash yellow rather than bright orange. It will, however, be a brave food manufacturer that takes the lead in omitting colours from all foods. The E numbers for colorants range from E100 to E180.

## Emulsifiers and stabilisers

Emulsifiers enable oils and fats to mix with water in foods. Stabilisers prevent them from separating again. They are needed in foods like mayonnaise and fat spreads. This group also includes thickeners such as guar gum and carrageen. Their E numbers range from E400 to E495.

## Flavourings

Most natural flavours are as harmless as the food whose flavour they mimic. The flavourings that generate concern on health grounds tend to be the chemical, non-caloric sweeteners, such as cyclamate, now banned in the UK because of evidence that it was possibly associated with cancer when taken in high concentrations. People with the genetic disease phenylketonuria must avoid aspartame because it is based on the amino acid phenylalanine, which they are unable to metabolise. However, weighing up the evidence for and against the use of sugars versus sweeteners, sugar is potentially capable of more damage to health than any of the permitted sweeteners.

## *Some additives that cause concern*

**Tartrazine (E102):** a yellow colouring; may cause allergic reactions in susceptible people.

**Azo-dyes and coal tar dyes:** thought by a few to cause behavioural problems, notably hyperactivity in children.

**Benzoic acid (E210):** a preservative; may cause gastric irritation.

**Nitrates and nitrites (E249–E252):** preservatives used in curing meats such as bacon, ham and corned beef. They have been associated with cancer when consumed in large amounts; they are banned from baby foods.

**Gallates (E310–E312):** antioxidants which can cause gastric irritation. They are not permitted in baby foods.

**Butylated-hydroxyanisole (BHA) and butylated hydroxy-toluene (BHT) (E320 and E321):** antioxidants which, in high doses, have caused cancers in rats. Closely related to gallates, they can also cause gastric irritation.

**Monosodium glutamate (E621):** a flavour enhancer, MSG can cause adverse effects when consumed in large amounts.

## Additive-induced hyperactivity

The conclusions of three separate studies on hyperactivity in children suggest that far fewer children suffer from additive-induced hyperactivity than parents believe. None denied that there may be a very small number who could be affected, but these were a tiny minority. The studies also pointed out that it was unfair to children to put them on a restrictive diet unless it was proven that additives were the cause of their hyperactivity. In fact, where children had been found to be sensitive to some foods, the foods had been from a variety of 'natural' food such as cow's milk, oranges or wheat. That said, many parents are convinced that eliminating certain additives does work, and the Hyperactive Children's Support Group regards food sensitivity as a major cause of hyperactivity. It has a list of 23 additives that it recommends should be avoided; of these, 16 are colorants.

# ———— Food irradiation ————

Food irradiation is now permitted as a method of food preservation in the UK, along with at least 36 other countries. By law, all foods that have undergone radiation must be labelled as such.

Initial public fears that irradiation could induce radioactivity in the food itself have proved unsubstantiated. Over the past 20 years, many hundreds of animal experiments using irradiated foods have failed to show any adverse effects when recommendations by regulatory bodies on the strength and type of applied radiation have been followed. It is claimed that no other food processing method has been the subject of such close scrutiny and that the conclusion must be that the process is at least as safe as any of the more traditional processes used by food manufacturers.

Some foods react better to irradiation than others, and detrimental changes can occur in texture, taste and colour. Meat, eggs and dairy products, for instance, do not generally respond well to irradiation. All this means is that the use of irradiation is limited to certain foods which respond well.

Food irradiation has an effect similar to a very gentle method of heat pasteurisation – so gentle that it is almost impossible to distinguish between irradiated and unirradiated foods. One of the criticisms levelled at food irradiation is that it allows unscrupulous food processors to utilise foods that are on the borderline or are past their best. Irradiation cannot, in fact, correct food already spoiled, although some claim it can disguise it by, for instance, removing nasty odours. Neither can irradiation make good food previously made dangerous by toxin-producing micro-organisms. It cannot be used to cover up for poor food hygiene or as a substitute for good manufacturing practice.

As with other forms of processing, some deterioration in nutrient content must be expected with irradiation. These losses in certain instances compare favourably with other methods of food preservation.

Food irradiation has proved particularly advantageous in processing herbs and spices. Under normal circumstances, these can carry bacteria which may contaminate the host food in which they are used. If the herbs and spices were heat-treated to destroy the bacteria, it would also destroy the flavours. The present preferred method of treatment is with gases, such as methyl bromide, but these are themselves the subject of regulation. Irradiation in this case eliminates the need for chemical treatment in removing the hygiene hazard and at the same time allows the flavours which are their functional purpose to be retained. In low doses, it is also very effective at inhibiting the sprouting of potatoes, killing insects in grains and accelerating the ageing of flour to make it suitable for bread making.

In summary, the advantages in the controlled use of food irradiation, both for the manufacturer and for the consumer, outweigh the minor dis-advantage of nutrient losses, which are comparable with other current processing methods.

# 10
# FOOD LABELLING

## Food labels

Historically, food manufacturers have always been reluctant to disclose what ingredients they use in their products, mainly because the information was potentially useful to their competitors, but perhaps also because they did not want to divulge the less wholesome ways in which they may have been adulterating or adding bulk to their foods.

There are now many regulations which govern how foods must be labelled, relating to the name, description, ingredients, datemarks and nutritional content.

### Name and description

The name of a product must say what the food is; it must not be misleading and it must state if it has been processed in some way, e.g. heat treated (UHT), dried or smoked.

### Weight

The weight, usually in grams (g) or millilitres (ml), is useful when looking for the best value for money against other similar products. The 'e' which follows the weight of the product means that the average quantity must be accurate, but the weight of each pack may vary slightly.

## Ingredients

Packaged foods must have a complete list of ingredients, listed in decreasing order of weight, including most food additives. The latter may be listed by name, such as ascorbic acid, by UK number or by E number (indicating EC approval) and should be preceded by a description of their function, for example colour, preservative or emulsifier. Labels must say if flavourings have been used but do not have to say what they are.

Food that is sold unwrapped, such as fresh-baked bread or food from a delicatessen counter, does not have to have a list of ingredients, but a ticket must be displayed near the food which shows its proper name and the type of ingredients, including whether it contains, for instance, preservatives.

## Datemarks

The term 'sell by' was phased out in 1990 because it was not clear to the consumer when the product had to be eaten by. The terms 'use by' and 'best before' are now the terms used instead.

Since 1 April 1991, it has been an offence to sell food after its 'use by' date. The options to the consumer who has a chilled meat pie or other chilled convenience food in the fridge is to eat it, cook it, freeze it or throw it away.

Most foods that can be safely kept for a little longer carry a 'best before' date. These foods may not be dangerous but are simply, as they say, past their best.

Both 'use by' and 'best before' dates are made on the grounds that they have been subjected to correct storage (see pages 79–80 and 159–161) and are prepared according to the manufacturers' instructions.


## *Nutrition labelling*

Until 1992, food manufacturers were free to give nutrition information on their labels in different ways and in different formats, but a new EC directive has been brought into force on nutrition labelling for packaged foods in specific formats.

The directive is considered by some experts to be weak, since it has not called for compulsory labelling of all foods. Instead, the only situation where nutrition labelling is compulsory is when a claim such as 'low in fat' or 'high fibre' is made. If no claim is made, labelling will remain optional. If nutrition labelling is adopted, then the format must be based either on:

- Group 1: the 'Big Four', i.e. kilocalories, protein, fat and carbo-hydrate;
- Group 2: the 'Big Four' plus the 'Little Four', i.e. kilocalories, protein, fat and carbohydrate plus saturated fat, sugar, fibre and sodium.

Where a nutrition claim is made for sugars, saturated fat, fibre or sodium, the information must contain those nutrients in Group 2. Information should be expressed per 100g (3.5oz) or per 100ml. It may, in addition, be given per serving, providing the number of portions contained in the packet is stated.

Declaration of other nutrients, such as the following, is optional.

- Amounts of fat as polyunsaturates, monounsaturates and cho-lesterol, as long as the amount of saturated fat is also stated.
- Amounts of carbohydrate as polyols and starch, as well as sugars.
- Vitamins and minerals, as set out in the table below, may be listed only when present in significant amounts, i.e. as a general rule, when 15 per cent or more of the recommended daily amount is supplied by 100g or per portion. These must also be expressed as a percentage of the recommended daily intake, provided the information relates to the food as prepared for consumption.

| Vitamin A | mcg | 800 | Vitamin B12 | mcg | 1 |
|---|---|---|---|---|---|
| Vitamin D | mcg | 5 | Biotin | mg | 0.15 |
| Vitamin E | mg | 10 | Pantothenic acid | mg | 6 |
| Vitamin C | mg | 60 | Calcium | mg | 800 |
| Thiamin | mg | 1.4 | Phosphorus | mg | 800 |
| Riboflavin | mg | 1.6 | Iron | mg | 14 |
| Niacin | mg | 18 | Magnesium | mg | 300 |
| Vitamin B6 | mg | 2 | Zinc | mg | 15 |
| Folic acid | mcg | 200 | Iodine | mcg | 150 |

Vitamins and minerals which may be declared and their recommended daily intakes (EC Council Directive (90/496/EEC))

## How to use nutrition labelling

The main aim of nutrition labelling is to provide the consumer with information about the nutrient content of the foods they eat. Potentially, it can give the consumer control over the nutritional quality of what he or she eats, but this can only happen if the consumer understands the basic principles of healthy eating and knows what to look for. To say a product contains 54g of fat per 100g of food, as in the case of peanut butter, can mean very little unless you know what the recommended intake of fat is (approximately 70g per day for women and 95g for men). If that food is normally only eaten in small amounts then, to have it as part of a varied diet is fine, but if 100g were eaten at a time, then clearly that person's total fat intake is likely to be too high. The 'average' recommended amount per day is given below for fat, saturated fat, fibre as non-starch polysaccharides and added sugar as non-milk extrinsic sugars.

| | Recom- mended intake* | Men | Women |
|---|---|---|---|
| Kcals (per day) | | 2,550 | 1,940 |
| Total fat | 33% of kcals | Not more than: 94g | 71g |
| Saturated fat | 10% of kcals | Not more than: 28g | 22g |
| Fibre (NSP) | g per day | Average: 18g | 18g (Range 12–24g) |
| Added sugar (NME) | 10% of kcals | Not more than: 68g | 52g |

How much per day? – A ready reckoner
Crown copyright. Reproduced by permission of the Controller of HMSO.

## Comparing nutrition information

Nutrition labelling is also very useful for comparing the contents of one brand or variety of a food with another. For example, how much more fibre or less sugar does Shredded Wheat have compared to cornflakes? How much less fat and saturated fat does a 'low fat' sausage contain compared to what one normally buys? If I have four slices of a wholemeal loaf a day, how much more fibre will I consume compared to four slices of white bread?

## Regulation of nutrition claims

A nutrition claim means any representation or advertising message which states, suggests or implies that a foodstuff has particular nutrition properties due to the energy or nutrients it contains.

Nutrition claims range from the general, such as 'healthy', to the specific, such as 'helps lower cholesterol'. They can be:

- Misleading: to call a low fat spread 'low fat' may mean it has half the fat of butter or margarine but, with about 40g fat per 100g, low fat spread is not a low fat food.
- Selective: for example, a breakfast cereal may state it is high in fibre at the same time as withholding information that it is also high in sugar.

Legislation for nutrition claims in the UK is therefore not sufficiently tight, but this is likely to change when a new directive, now being prepared by the European Commission, comes into force.

## Summary – what to look for on labels

- Choose products which have better quality ingredients, e.g. sunflower oil rather than 'vegetable fat', or the product with 'sugar' lower down the list of ingredients.
- Don't use foods that have passed their 'use by' dates.
- Make your own judgement about any claims, for example 'low fat', by reading the nutrition label.
- Compare nutrient values of similar products. The most important elements are kilocalories, fat and saturated fat.
- Use the weight to compare value for money with other products.

# 11

## MENU PLANNING
## AND
## CHOOSING FOOD

## ─────── Eating in ───────

### *Healthy eating in everyday life*

Eating means a lot more than nutrition – it means planning menus, buying food and preparing and serving it. Many considerations need to be taken into account, especially if you are cooking for others – will they like it, can I afford it, have I time to make it? With these in mind, let's recap on the current recommendations for healthy eating. In general, we should plan to eat:

- more fibre;
- more starchy foods;
- less fat, especially saturated fat;
- less sugar;
- less salt.

We should also:

- moderate alcohol intake;
- maintain ideal body weight.

### Eat more fibre

- Include more foods that come from plants: more vegetables, fresh fruit, cereals, pulses, nuts, wholemeal breads and high fibre cereals.

- Choose wholegrain alternatives to white or refined products, e.g. brown rice, wholemeal pasta, bread, rolls and breakfast cereals.
- Incorporate wholemeal flour into recipes, either using half wholemeal and half white flour or using all wholemeal.
- Bulk up stews and casseroles with pulses such as kidney beans, baked beans or chickpeas.
- Jacket potatoes in their skins make an excellent alternative to roast or chipped potatoes.

## Eat more starchy foods

- Eating a diet with more fibre will probably mean you are eating more starchy foods too. It is much better to eat white alternatives to wholemeal bread, pasta and rice than to eat neither because you don't like wholemeal.
- Slice bread more thickly for sandwiches and try eating bread the continental way, i.e. with meals but without butter or other fat spread.
- As you decrease the fat and sugar in your diet, replace the calories with more bread and larger portions of potato, other root vegetables, pasta and rice.
- Try new recipes based on pulses, rice and wholegrain cereals.

## Eat less fat

Over 60 per cent of the fat in our diet is from hidden sources such as milk, cheese, eggs, chocolate, biscuits, cakes and pastry. Although the aim is to cut down on the total amount of fat in our diet, priority should be given to reducing saturated fats, which mainly come from animal sources.

- Use low fat or semi-skimmed milk.
- Use yoghurt or fromage frais rather than cream.
- Buy lean meat and more fish.
- Cut down on high fat foods such as pastries, pies, fatty meats and meat products.
- Choose more low fat alternatives, such as low fat spreads, salad dressings, mayonnaises, low fat cheeses and low fat sausages.
- Choose low or medium fat cheeses instead of hard, full fat or cream cheeses.
- Use mashed potatoes as a topping to savoury dishes instead of pastry.
- Choose mixed fruit and nuts in preference to sweets, chocolate or crisps.

— 173 —

- Spread fat on one side of a sandwich only.
- Grill foods rather than fry them.
- For cooking, use an oil high in polyunsaturates, such as sunflower or corn.

## Eat less sugar

We tend to think of sugar as that white granular substance which is easily identifiable. However, sugar includes not only sucrose but also fructose, maltose, glucose (dextrose), honey, molasses, glucose syrup and brown sugars. None of these have any nutritional value other than supplying calories.

- Check label ingredients for less obvious forms of sugar.
- Buy breakfast cereals with a low sugar content (compare labels).
- Add less sugar to recipes.
- Use artificial sweeteners in hot drinks and stewed fruit or, better still, wean yourself off adding sugar to unsweetened hot drinks, cereals and fruits.
- Replace chocolate and sweets with fruit, fresh or dried.
- Choose tinned fruit canned in natural juice.
- Instead of buying fruit yoghurt, buy plain and add puréed or chopped fruit to it.
- Buy fewer biscuits and cakes.
- Choose 'diet' fizzy drinks and squashes.
- Choose low sugar versions of jams and marmalades.
- Have fresh fruit instead of puddings.

## Use less salt

- Eat fewer processed foods, including ham and bacon.
- Reduce the amount of salt in cooking.
- Don't add salt at the table.
- Use low salt alternatives where possible.
- Cut down on salty snack foods, such as salted nuts and crisps.
- Sea salt is no better health-wise than table salt.

## Planning for healthy changes

It is best to try to introduce changes gradually, maybe one or two changes every one or two weeks. If you decide to cut down on an item, say chocolate, compensate by having more fruit or an extra half a sandwich. Because you are cutting down on some foods, you will, unless overweight, need to eat more starchy foods such as potatoes, bread, rice and pasta. This will help prevent you feeling hungry and defeating the object by eating unhealthy snack foods to satisfy your hunger.

It may be helpful to write down a list of the meals you cook or prepare on a regular basis, and then consider whether they fit into a healthy eating plan or not; if not, can you adjust the recipe?

This may involve the substitution of certain foodstuffs, for example, low fat milk for whole milk, or using an oil high in polyunsaturates rather than a white cooking fat. It may involve changing cooking methods, for example, poaching or grilling rather than frying, or it may mean changes in preparation methods, such as eliminating the 'frying off' stage. These changes may be invisible to the consumer but they can make a substantial move towards achieving dietary goals without the introduction of unfamiliar foods. The table below illustrates how changing ingredients can alter the nutrient content.

|  | Method 1 | Method 2 | Method 3 |
|---|---|---|---|
| Ingredients | 100g butter 100g white flour 1 litre whole milk | 100g sunflower margarine 100g white flour 1 litre low fat milk | 50g sunflower margarine 50g white flour 50g wholemeal flour 1 litre low fat milk |
| Calories Fat (g) Saturated fat (g) Fibre (g) | 1,730 120 77 3.6 | 1,400 83 15 3.6 | 1,020 43 7.7 6.1 |

Nutrient analysis: white sauce per litre

## Healthy alternatives

There will probably be some recipes that simply don't lend themselves to healthy eating. Gradually try to introduce new recipes that can replace the less healthy ones. Here are some suggestions:

## Healthy breakfast suggestions

- Wholewheat breakfast cereals served with low fat or semi-skimmed milk.
- Porridge made with water, low fat or semi-skimmed milk.

- Home-made muesli with oats, dried and/or fresh chopped fruit and nuts served with low fat or semi-skimmed milk.
- Wholegrain toast, low fat spread and a boiled egg.
- Wholegrain toast, low fat spread and baked beans.
- Lean grilled bacon, grilled tomato and poached egg.
- Low fat yoghurt or fromage frais with chopped fresh fruit.
- Dried fruit, stewed, with fromage frais.
- Stewed apple topped with crumbled wholewheat breakfast cereal.
- Fresh-baked bread, preferably wholegrain, low fat spread, lean cold meats, sliced medium fat cheeses and fresh fruit.
- Poached kippers or haddock.

## Light meal suggestions

- Jacket potatoes with baked beans, stir-fried vegetables or chilli con carne (lean meat).
- Baked beans on toast.
- Grilled fish fingers, mashed potatoes and frozen peas.
- Tuna and pasta.
- Home-made vegetable soups with wholemeal French bread.
- Grated cheese grilled on toast with tomatoes on top.
- Lean meat/chicken (without skin) and salad.
- Smoked mackerel, sardines or pilchards and salad.
- Chicken risotto.
- Kedgeree and green salad.
- Spaghetti bolognaise.
- Home-made burger in a bun.
- Cauliflower cheese.
- Pizza and salad.
- Spanish omelette with peas, potatoes and mushrooms and wholemeal French bread.

## Packed lunch ideas

- Sandwiches
  **Bread:** Try making sandwiches with thick-cut bread, preferably wholemeal, granary or brown, but if you really prefer white, then choose white – it is still a healthy food.
  **Spread:** Whatever you use, spread it sparingly. Best choice if trying to keep fat intake down would be low fat spread, preferably made with sunflower, soya or other named oil.
  **Fillings:**
  (a)  Meat: turkey or chicken without skin, other lean meats.

(b) Cheese: low or medium fat cheeses such as Edam, Gouda, cottage or curd cheese with peppers, onion, celery or other vegetables.

(c) Fish: tinned fish such as tuna, sardines, pilchards, preferably tinned in brine or tomato juice rather than oil.

(d) Other: peanut butter and mashed banana.

Salads can be added to all the above fillings to provide variety and interest to your sandwiches, or simply have salad on its own as a sandwich filling.

- Salads
  (a) Rice, preferably brown, with ham, peppers, sweetcorn, tomato, mushrooms and/or chopped celery.
  (b) Pasta, preferably wholemeal, with tuna or tinned salmon and red pepper or other raw chopped vegetables.
  (c) Pizza, preferably home-made.
  (d) Chicken drumsticks.
- Flask of home-made soup and granary rolls.
- Unsalted peanuts and raisins.
- Home-made oatmeal and fruit biscuits.
- Natural yoghurt with chopped fruit added.
- Fresh fruit.
- Fresh juice.

## Main meal suggestions

- Liver and bacon casserole with jacket potato, peas and cabbage.
- Shepherd's pie made with 'extra lean' mince, green beans and carrots.
- Grilled lean meat, mashed potatoes, spring greens and grilled tomatoes.
- Grilled white fish, new potatoes, broccoli and green salad.
- Fish pie, courgettes and runner beans.
- Chicken tandoori, boiled rice with peppers and sweetcorn, mixed salad.
- Pasta with a tomato and prawn sauce.
- Roast chicken, stir-fried vegetables, jacket potato.
- Grilled trout, mashed potatoes, peas and grilled tomatoes.
- Curried chicken with brown rice and green salad.
- Mixed bean casserole and salad.
- Baked mackerel with gooseberry sauce, new potatoes, braised leeks.

# Eating out

Dining out healthily is easier than it used to be in many restaurants. A growing number now recognise the need to have alternative choices to dishes cooked in heavy sauces, vegetables swimming in butter and French fries with everything. A good chef can always provide a healthy choice without you having to sacrifice the pleasures of a good meal. Of course, there will be times when you won't want to think about calories or health, and the occasional indulgent meal will do no harm.

Takeaways, although very convenient, do tend to be high in fat and salt and low in fibre although there are exceptions, such as shish kebab with salad and pitta bread, and jacket potatoes with low fat fillings.

Healthy eating when dining out starts with your choice of restaurant. For instance, seafood restaurants and Japanese restaurants will usually have a good choice of fish without rich sauces and without being fried.

Good choices when eating out include:

**Starters:** grapefruit; melon; soup, either clear or a non-cream variety; smoked fish such as salmon, trout or mackerel; seafood salad without dressing; moules marinière; mushrooms or other vegetables à la Grecque; pasta with a tomato or other non-cream-based sauce.

**Main courses:** any lean roast or grilled meat dish served without fatty sauces; fish grilled, poached or steamed without cream-based sauces; pasta without cream-based sauces; vegetable dishes without added fat; salad dishes without rich dressings; jacket or boiled potatoes.

**Sweet course:** fresh fruit salad; sorbets; fruit marinated in liqueur; fruit compôte; summer pudding.

**Indian:** best to choose dishes that are not in oily sauces, for example tandoori and tikka dishes. Naan bread, chapatis, plain or pilau rice, dhal and raita are all healthy choices.

**Chinese:** Chinese food can be very healthy, although it tends to be rather high in monosodium glutamate. It is best to avoid fried dishes, such as spring rolls, sweet and sour dishes and fried rice; most other dishes are usually relatively low in fat.

**Italian:** pasta with a tomato or other vegetable-based sauce; pizzas with salad; fish, chicken or lean meat dishes cooked with very little or no oil or butter; salads and vegetables without fat.

# — FURTHER READING —

DHSS *Catering for Health: The Recipe File*, HSMO, 1988
Marshall, J. & Heughan, A. *Eat for Life Diet*, Vermilion, 1992
Poulter, J. *Healthy Eating in the Workplace*, HEA, 1994
Robins, C. *The Healthy Catering Manual*, Dorling Kindersley, 1989
Silverstone, R. *Healthy Eating: A Guide for Chefs and Caterers*, McMillan, 1990
Stevenson, D. *Basic Cookery: The Process Approach*, Stanley Thornes, 1991
Stevenson, D. & Scobie, P. *Catering for Health*, Hutchinson, 1987
*The Open University Guide to Healthy Eating*, Rambletree Pelham, 1985

# GLOSSARY

**Aflatoxins:** Aflatoxin is a mould that grows on peanuts and grains if stored in moist, warm conditions after harvesting. It can cause liver damage, and possibly cancer of the liver. Avoid eating nuts that are obviously mouldy or decayed.

**Antibodies:** Antibodies are protein molecules formed in response to invasion of foreign organisms such as viruses. They play an important part in the body's natural defence mechanism. Any substance that causes the body to produce antibodies is called an antigen. The cells responsible for making antibodies are the white blood cells.

**Antioxidants:** Antioxidants are part of the body's defence mechanism against free radicals. They neutralise them by donating the missing part to the free radicals without becoming unstable themselves. Antioxidant nutrients exert protective effects against several diseases and play an important role in the body's defence systems. The antioxidant vitamins include vitamin A, its precursor carotene, and vitamins C and E. Antioxidant minerals include iron, zinc, copper and selenium.

**Aspartame:** Aspartame is an artificial sweetener made from the amino acid, phenylalanine. It tastes like sugar but is much sweeter. As a protein, it provides 4 kilocalories per gram, but because so little is used, it is almost calorie free. It has largely replaced saccharin as the low calorie sweetener of choice in many commercial diet drinks and other low calorie products. It is very acceptable for use in drinks and cold puddings but is unsuitable for baking or cooking. Aspartame is unsuitable for individuals with the disease phenylketonuria.

**Bacteria:** Bacteria are single-cell organisms, making them one of the simplest forms of life. Most species of bacteria are not harmful to man, and many perform useful functions. For example, bacteria help to ferment milk and are necessary for making yoghurt and for ripening cheese. Some bacteria are, however, harmful, causing food contamination. The most common form of food poisoning in the home is caused by the contamination of food with the bacteria salmonella. They can also cause many serious diseases, including tuberculosis, diphtheria, typhoid and pneumonia.

**Beta-carotene:** The origin of vitamin A is a group of components called carotenoids, of which beta-carotene is the most active. It is a yellow pigment found in plants, particularly those with yellow, red and dark green colouring. Animals, including humans, can convert the beta-carotene of their food into vitamin A. There is growing evidence that a high intake of foods containing beta-carotene may protect against certain cancers including lung and prostate cancer.

**Caffeine:** Caffeine is the main physiologically active ingredient in coffee and it is also found in tea, cola seeds and cola fruit. It is a natural stimulant and acts on the central nervous system, increasing alertness and concentration. Caffeine, although a drug, seems to be relatively harmless in moderate amounts for healthy adults. In large amounts it can produce a reaction similar to that caused by anxiety. Like some other drugs, caffeine can be addictive, and withdrawal or changing to a decaffeinated alternative can cause headaches characteristic of withdrawal symptoms. There seems to be no conclusive evidence that a moderate consumption of caffeine during pregnancy is a hazard to the unborn baby.

**Complex carbohydrates:** These are starchy, fibrous foods including cereals, bread, pasta, rice, potatoes, pulses, whole grains, vegetables and fruit.

**Cyclamate:** Cyclamate is a sweetening agent, 30 times as sweet as sucrose (sugar). It was banned in 1976 in the UK, the USA and other countries because some animals developed cancer following regular very high doses of it.

**Electrolytes:** Electrolytes are formed when mineral salts dissolve in water and separate into negatively and positively charged ions. The body uses these electrolytes to help regulate the distribution and composition of its fluids. This is vital to all cells, which must be constantly bathed in fluid both inside and outside the cell walls.

**Enzymes:** Enzymes are biological catalysts which enable specific reactions to take place in our body. They facilitate chemical reactions to take place without themselves being changed in the process. Digestive enzymes help to decompose food for use by the body.

**Essential fatty acids (EFAs):** Two polyunsaturated fatty acids have been designated as essential fatty acids: linoleic acid and alpha-linolenic acid. They cannot be synthesised by the body and have to be obtained from the food we eat. They have important roles in maintaining the integrity of cell membranes. Serum cholesterol has been shown to be lowered by essential fatty acids, particularly linoleic acid. The EFAs are also precursors of a group of hormone-like substances that help to regulate blood pressure, heart rate, blood clotting and the central nervous system.

**Free radicals:** Free radicals are unstable molecules which have part of their structure missing and try to replace it from other molecules. In doing so, they are capable of damaging other cells and could be a starting point for some cancers and for the deposition of cholesterol in the arteries.

**Ginseng:** Ginseng is a plant whose extract has been inappropriately promoted as an energy-giving aid, when in fact no products impart such a quality. Side effects of chronic use include nervousness, confusion and depression.

**Hormones:** Hormones help to regulate chemical processes that go in the body. They are generated in specific organs such as the thyroid gland. Thyroid hormones affect growth in childhood and they control the rate at which our bodies use up nutrients, i.e. the metabolic rate. Other hormones include adrenalin which prepares the body for action under stressful situations, insulin which helps to regulate blood sugar levels, the sex hormones, testosterone which stimulates sex characteristics in men, and oestrogen and progesterone in women. Some hormones are used as medicines, often simply to treat deficiencies such as insulin for diabetics and hormone replacement therapy (HRT) for women suffering symptoms of the menopause. Other examples include the contraceptive pill and corticosteroids, which are used to treat inflammatory diseases such as rheumatoid arthritis and asthma.

**Lecithin:** Lecithin is a phospholipid containing glycerol, fatty acids, phosphoric acid and choline and is widely distributed in foods, although liver, egg yolk and soyabeans are especially rich sources. Although promoted as a health food, lecithin is not absorbed as such from the digestive tract but is broken down into its constituent fatty acids, choline, etc. The lecithin needed for building cell membranes and other functions is made by the liver and not obtained from food or supplements.

**Metabolism:** Metabolism has been called the 'fire of life', and food provides its fuel. It is the process by which the body converts nutrients from food into useful energy which can be used for performance of work and for synthesising compounds which are vital for cellular structure and function. It is an ongoing process in every cell in the body, requiring a continuous supply of nutrients.

**Metabolic rate:** The basal metabolic rate is the amount of energy used when the body is fasting and at complete rest. It indicates the amount of energy needed to sustain life processes – respiration, circulation, glandular activity, metabolism and maintenance of body temperature. The thyroid gland is the principal regulator of metabolic rate. If the thyroid gland is overactive, the basal metabolic rate may increase by almost twice the normal rate. Conversely, if it is underactive, basal metabolism may fall by as much as 50 per cent. Women have a 5–10 per cent lower metabolic rate than men, and a tall thin person has a higher metabolic rate than a short fat person because they have a larger surface area in which to lose heat.

**Monosodium glutamate:** Monosodium glutamate is a flavour enhancer commonly used in Chinese cooking. It has received publicity because some individuals appear to have an adverse reaction to it, including facial flushing, throbbing headaches and, in severe cases, heart palpitations and vomiting. It is found in large amounts in soya sauce.

**Phospholipid:** Any lipid containing phosphorus is included in the category of phospholipid. They are found in every cell in the body and help to maintain the structural integrity of the cell. The best known phospholipid is lecithin.

**Pica:** Pica is an unnatural craving for substances that have little or no nutritional value.

**Precursor:** The term precursor is used to describe a parent or source compound; for example beta-carotene is a precursor of vitamin A, and the parent n-6 polyunsaturated fatty acid, linoleic acid, is the precursor of arachidonic acid.

**Sorbitol:** Sorbitol is a sweetener derived from glucose. It is absorbed slowly and for this reason has a place in diabetic products such as diabetic chocolate and preserves. It does contribute to calorie intake and is so is not suitable for use in a calorie-restricted diet. In large amounts, it can cause diarrhoea.

# — APPENDICES —

## — Weight equivalents —

| | | |
|---:|:---:|:---|
| 28g | = | 1oz |
| 56g | = | 2oz |
| 85g | = | 3oz |
| 112g | = | 4oz |
| 140g | = | 5oz |
| 170g | = | 6oz |
| 200g | = | 7oz |
| 225g | = | 8oz |
| 250g | = | 9oz |
| 285g | = | 10oz |

# APPENDIX 1

## Calorie contents of some commonly eaten foods, per average serving

|  | *Calories* |
|---|---:|
| **Bread and Cereal Products** | |
| bread, white, 1 slice, 40g | 94 |
| wholemeal, 1 slice, 40g | 86 |
| roll, 1 crusty, 50g | 140 |
| biscuit, arrowroot, 7g | 32 |
| cream cracker, 7g | 30 |
| digestive, 17g | 80 |
| shortbread, 15g | 70 |
| cake, fruitcake, 90g | 320 |
| Danish pastry, 110g | 410 |
| doughnut, 75g | 300 |
| pizza, 200g | 470 |
| rice, boiled, 150g | 210 |
| spaghetti, boiled, 230g | 240 |
| **Fats and oil** | |
| butter, average spread, 10g | 74 |
| margarine, average spread, 10g | 74 |
| low fat spread (40% fat), 10g | 37 |
| oil, vegetable, 2tsp, 10ml | 90 |

| **Dairy products** | See Appendix 3 |
|---|---|

| **Meat and meat products** | See Appendix 2 |
|---|---|

| **Fish** | See Appendix 2 |
|---|---|

## Vegetables

| | |
|---|---|
| baked beans, 135g | 113 |
| broccoli, 90g | 22 |
| brussels sprouts, 90g | 32 |
| cabbage, 90g | 14 |
| carrots, 90g | 22 |
| mushrooms, fried, 45g | 71 |
| peas, frozen, boiled, 90g | 62 |
| potatoes, boiled, 200g | 144 |
| potatoes, roast, 200g | 298 |
| potatoes, chipped, 200g | 478 |
| potato crisps, 1 bag, 25g | 136 |
| tomato, raw, 90g | 15 |
| tomato, fried, 90g | 82 |

## Fruit (weight without skin or stone)

| | |
|---|---|
| apple, 1 medium, 112g | 53 |
| avocado pear, ½ medium, 75g | 142 |
| banana, 1 medium, 100g | 95 |
| orange, 1 medium, 160g | 60 |
| peach, 1 medium, 110g | 36 |
| strawberries, 112g | 30 |

## Nuts (weight without shell)

| | |
|---|---|
| almonds, 6 whole, 10g | 61 |
| chestnuts, 1 whole, 10g | 17 |
| peanuts, roasted, 10 whole, 10g | 60 |

## Soft drinks

| | |
|---|---|
| lemonade, 1 can, 330ml | 70 |
| cola, 1 can, 330ml | 130 |
| orange juice, fresh, 1 glass, 200ml | 72 |
| tomato juice, 1 glass, 200ml | 28 |

## Sugar and preserves

| | |
|---|---:|
| honey, 1 average spread, 20g | 58 |
| jam, 1 average spread, 15g | 39 |
| marmalade, 1 average spread, 15g | 39 |
| sugar, 1tsp, 5g | 20 |

## Alcohol

| | |
|---|---:|
| bitter, draught, ½ pint | 90 |
| lager, bottled, ½ pint | 82 |
| stout, bottled, ½ pint | 105 |
| cider, dry, ½ pint | 102 |
| wine, dry white, 1 glass, 125ml | 83 |
| wine, medium white, 1 glass, 125ml | 94 |
| wine, red, 1 glass, 125ml | 85 |
| spirits, 1 pub measure, 24ml | 53 |

Data/information from *The Composition of Foods*, 5th ed. (1991) is reproduced with the permission of the Royal Society of Chemistry and the Controller of HMSO.

# APPENDIX 2

## Calorie, fat and saturated fat contents of meat, poultry and fish per serving

| Food | Calories | Total fat (grams) | Saturated fat (grams) |
|---|---|---|---|
| **Meat and meat products** | | | |
| **Bacon** | | | |
| 1 rasher, grilled, lean only, 25g | 73 | 4.7 | 1.9 |
| 1 rasher, back, grilled, lean and fat, 25g | 101 | 8.5 | 3.3 |
| **Beef** | | | |
| topside, roast, lean only, 100g | 156 | 4.4 | 1.4 |
| topside, roast, lean and fat, 100g | 214 | 12.0 | 4.1 |
| **Poultry** | | | |
| chicken, roast, no skin, 100g | 148 | 5.4 | 1.6 |
| chicken, roast, meat and skin, 100g | 216 | 14.0 | 4.2 |
| duck, roast, meat and skin, 100g | 339 | 29.0 | 7.9 |
| **Lamb** | | | |
| leg, roast, lean only, 100g | 191 | 8.1 | 3.9 |
| shoulder, roast, lean and fat, 100g | 316 | 26.3 | 13.1 |

## Pork

| | | | |
|---|---|---|---|
| chop, grilled, lean only, 100g | 226 | 10.7 | 3.8 |
| leg, roast, lean and fat, 100g | 286 | 19.8 | 7.3 |
| leg, roast, lean only, 100g | 185 | 6.9 | 2.4 |

## Offal

| | | | |
|---|---|---|---|
| liver, lamb's, fried, 100g | 232 | 14.0 | 4.0 |

## Other meat products

| | | | |
|---|---|---|---|
| corned beef | 217 | 12.1 | 6.3 |
| ham, tinned, 100g | 120 | 5.1 | 1.9 |
| liver sausage, 100g | 310 | 26.9 | 7.9 |
| pork pie, individual, 140g | 526 | 37.8 | 14.3 |
| sausages, pork, grilled, 1 large, 60g | 191 | 14.8 | 5.7 |
| sausage roll, 1 medium, 60g | 286 | 21.8 | 8.0 |
| steak & kidney pie, individual, 200g | 646 | 42.4 | 16.8 |

## *Fish and fish products*

### White fish

| | | | |
|---|---|---|---|
| cod, poached, medium portion, 120g | 113 | 1.3 | 0.5 |
| cod, fried in batter in veg. oil, 180g | 358 | 18.5 | 1.6 |
| cod, fried in batter in lard, 180g | 358 | 18.5 | 8.5 |

### Oily fish

| | | | |
|---|---|---|---|
| herring, grilled, 1 medium, 120g | 240 | 15.6 | 4.4 |
| mackerel, smoked, 1 medium, 150g | 531 | 46.3 | 9.4 |
| pilchards, td in tomato sauce, 100g | 126 | 5.4 | 1.1 |
| salmon, tinned, 100g | 155 | 8.2 | 1.5 |
| sardines, tinned in oil, drained, 100g | 217 | 13.6 | 2.8 |
| trout, brown, steamed, 1 average, 180g | 160 | 5.4 | 1.3 |
| tuna, tinned in brine, 100g | 99 | 0.6 | 0.2 |
| tuna, tinned in oil, drained, 100g | 189 | 9.0 | 1.4 |

### Shell fish (weight without shell)

| | | | |
|---|---|---|---|
| prawns, boiled, 56g | 60 | 1.0 | 0.2 |
| scampi, fried in veg. oil, 150g | 474 | 26.4 | 2.5 |

### Fish products

| | | | |
|---|---|---|---|
| fish fingers, 2 grilled, 56g | 120 | 5.0 | 1.6 |
| taramasalata, 1tbs/45g | 200 | 20.9 | 1.4 |

Data/information derived from *The Composition of Foods*, 5th ed. (1991) is reproduced with the permission of the Royal Society of Chemistry and the Controller of HMSO.

# ─── APPENDIX 3 ───

## ─ Calorie, fat and saturated fat contents of dairy products and eggs, per serving ─

| Food | Calories | Total fat (grams) | Saturated fat (grams) |
|---|---|---|---|
| **Milk (per half pint, 285ml)** | | | |
| full fat | 188 | 11.1 | 6.8 |
| semi-skimmed | 131 | 4.6 | 2.8 |
| skimmed | 94 | 0.3 | 0.3 |
| **Cream per 142ml/5oz carton** | | | |
| double | 638 | 68.2 | 42.6 |
| whipping | 530 | 55.8 | 34.9 |
| single | 281 | 27.1 | 16.9 |
| **Cheese per 50g serving** | | | |
| cream | 220 | 23.7 | 14.9 |
| Stilton | 206 | 17.8 | 11.1 |
| Cheddar type | 206 | 17.2 | 10.9 |
| Danish Blue type | 174 | 14.8 | 9.2 |
| Brie | 160 | 13.5 | 8.4 |
| Edam | 166 | 12.7 | 8.0 |
| reduced fat hard, e.g. Tendale | 130 | 7.5 | 4.7 |
| cottage | 49 | 2.0 | 1.2 |
| fromage frais, very low fat | 29 | 0.1 | 0.1 |

## Egg per size 2 egg

| | | | |
|---|---|---|---|
| boiled | 88 | 6.5 | 1.9 |
| fried in veg. oil | 107 | 8.3 | 2.4 |

## Yoghurt per 150g carton

| | | | |
|---|---|---|---|
| Greek | 172 | 13.6 | 7.8 |
| fruit | 135 | 1.0 | 0.6 |
| low fat natural | 84 | 1.2 | 0.7 |

Data/information from *The Composition of Foods*, 5th ed. (1991) is reproduced with the permission of the Royal Society of Chemistry and the Controller of HMSO.

# — APPENDIX 4 —

## Non-starch polysaccharide content of different foods, per 100g of food as eaten

| Food | Total NSP per 100g of food |
|---|---|
| **Breakfast cereals** | |
| Allbran | 24.5 |
| Branflakes | 13.0 |
| Shredded Wheat | 9.8 |
| Weetabix | 9.7 |
| muesli | 6.4 |
| Puffed wheat | 5.6 |
| Special K | 2.0 |
| Cornflakes | 0.9 |
| Rice Krispies | 0.7 |
| **Bread** | |
| wholemeal | 5.8 |
| granary | 4.3 |
| brown | 3.5 |
| white | 1.5 |

## Biscuits

| | |
|---|---|
| crispbread, rye | 11.7 |
| crackers, wholemeal | 4.4 |
| digestive | 2.2 |
| cream crackers | 2.2 |
| gingernuts | 1.4 |

## Other cereals

| | |
|---|---|
| spaghetti, wholemeal, boiled | 3.5 |
| spaghetti, white, boiled | 1.2 |
| rice, brown, boiled | 0.8 |
| rice, white, boiled | 0.1 |

## Vegetables

| | |
|---|---|
| beans, red kidney, boiled | 6.7 |
| beans, broad, boiled | 6.5 |
| peas, frozen, boiled | 5.1 |
| chickpeas, boiled | 4.3 |
| lentils, green, boiled | 3.8 |
| beans, baked | 3.7 |
| brussels sprouts, boiled | 3.1 |
| potatoes, jacket, with skin | 2.7 |
| carrots, boiled | 2.5 |
| lentils, red, boiled | 1.9 |
| cabbage, boiled | 1.8 |
| potatoes, boiled | 1.2 |

## Fruit and nuts

| | |
|---|---|
| apricots, dried, ready-to-eat | 6.3 |
| peanuts, roasted | 6.0 |
| raspberries | 2.5 |
| apples | 1.8 |
| oranges | 1.7 |
| bananas | 1.1 |

Data/information from *The Composition of Foods*, 5th ed. (1991) is reproduced with the permission of the Royal Society of Chemistry and the Controller of HMSO.

# APPENDIX 5

## Vitamins, their functions and deficiency symptoms

| Vitamin | Function | Deficiency symptom |
|---|---|---|
| Vitamin A | Essential for normal growth, healthy eyes and night vision, maintenance of healthy skin and mucous membranes and immune responses. | Increased susceptibility to bacterial infection. Skin changes, night blindness |
| Vitamin B1 | Controls conversion of carbohydrate foods to energy. Essential for growth, normal appetite, digestion and healthy nerves. | Mental confusion, muscle fatigue, emotional instability, depression, loss of appetite, beri-beri |
| Vitamin B2 | Essential for growth, health of eyes and for digestion. Involved in formation of thyroid enzyme regulating activities. | Soreness of lips, mouth and tongue; loss of visual acuity |

| | | |
|---|---|---|
| **Vitamin B3** | Helps to control the release of energy from protein, fat and carbohydrate, i.e. the three main components that make up food. | Muscular weakness, loss of appetite, indigestion, nausea, irritability, change in skin lesions, pellagra (dermatitis, dementia, diarrhoea) |
| **Vitamin B6** | Required for metabolism of protein (meat, fish, eggs, etc). Essential in formation of sheath surrounding nerve cells. Involved in immune system. | Depression, nausea, irritability, change in alertness |
| **Vitamin B12** | Essential for normal functioning of all body cells, especially for those of the nervous system and bone marrow. Promotes production of red blood cells. | Pernicious anaemia, degeneration of nerve endings |
| **Folic acid** | Essential for formation of red and white blood cells in bone marrow, and for their maturation. | Poor growth, anaemia and other blood disorders |
| **Vitamin C** | Multiple functions involved at enzyme level. Essential in formation of collagen in fibrous tissues such as cartilage, connective tissue and skin. Promotes healing of wounds, fractures and bleeding gums. Reduces liability to infection. | Poor appetite and growth, anaemia, inflamed gums, failure of wounds to heal, depression |
| **Vitamin D** | Essential for growth and development of bones and teeth. Important role in maintaining appropriate levels of calcium and phosphorus in the blood to support mineralisation of bones. | Fragility of bones, rickets in children |
| **Vitamin E** | Not yet fully understood. Appears to protect cell membranes from deterioration. | Muscle weakness |

# APPENDIX 6

## Estimated Average Requirements (EARs) for energy, fat, saturated fat and sugar (non-milk extrinsic sugars) per day

|  | Males | | | | | Females | | | | |
|---|---|---|---|---|---|---|---|---|---|---|
|  | kcals | fat (g) | saturated fat (g) | sugar (NME) (g) | fibre (NSP) (g) | kcals | fat (g) | saturated fat (g) | sugar (NME) (g) | fibre (NSP) (g) |
| 1–3 years | 1,230 | 45 | 14 | 33 | (i) | 1,165 | 43 | 13 | 31 | (i) |
| 4–6 years | 1,715 | 63 | 19 | 46 | (i) | 1,545 | 57 | 17 | 41 | (i) |
| 7–10 years | 1,970 | 72 | 22 | 53 | (i) | 1,740 | 64 | 19 | 46 | (i) |

| | | | | | | | | | |
|---|---|---|---|---|---|---|---|---|---|
| 11–14 years | 2,220 | 81 | 25 | 59 | 18 | 1,845 | 68 | 21 | 49 | 18 |
| 15–18 years | 2,755 | 101 | 31 | 73 | 18 | 2,110 | 77 | 23 | 56 | 18 |
| 19–50 years | 2,550 | 94 | 28 | 68 | 18 | 1,940 | 71 | 22 | 52 | 18 |
| 51–59 years | 2,550 | 94 | 28 | 68 | 18 | 1,900 | 70 | 21 | 51 | 18 |
| 60–64 years | 2,380 | 87 | 26 | 63 | 18 | 1,900 | 70 | 21 | 51 | 18 |
| 65–74 years | 2,330 | 85 | 26 | 62 | 18 | 1,900 | 70 | 21 | 51 | 18 |
| 75+ years | 2,100 | 77 | 23 | 56 | 18 | 1,810 | 66 | 20 | 48 | 18 |

Fat based on 33 per cent of total energy intake.
Saturated fat based on 10 per cent of total energy intake.
Non-milk extrinsic sugar based on 10 per cent of total energy intake.

(i) It is recommended that children should have proportionately less non-starch polysaccharides and that children of less than two years should not take foods rich in NSP at the expense of more energy-rich foods, required for adequate growth.

From: *Dietary Reference Values for Food Energy and Nutrients for the United Kingdom*, HMSO, London (1991). Reproduced with the permission of the Controller, HMSO.

# APPENDIX 7

## Reference Nutrient Intakes (RNIs) per day for selected nutrients

| Males | Protein (g) | Vit. B1 (mg) | Vit. B2 (mg) | Niacin (mg) | Vit. B6 (mg) | Vit. B12 (mcg) | Folate (mcg) | Vit. C (mg) | Vit. A (mcg) | Calcium (mg) | Iron (mg) | Zinc (mg) |
|---|---|---|---|---|---|---|---|---|---|---|---|---|
| 1–3 years | 14.5 | 0.5 | 0.6 | 8 | 0.7 | 0.5 | 70 | 30 | 400 | 350 | 6.9 | 5.0 |
| 4–6 years | 19.7 | 0.7 | 0.8 | 11 | 0.9 | 0.8 | 100 | 30 | 500 | 450 | 6.1 | 6.5 |
| 7–10 years | 28.3 | 0.7 | 1.0 | 12 | 1.0 | 1.0 | 150 | 30 | 500 | 550 | 8.7 | 7.0 |
| 11–14 years | 42.1 | 0.9 | 1.2 | 15 | 1.2 | 1.2 | 200 | 35 | 600 | 1,000 | 11.3 | 9.0 |
| 15–18 years | 55.2 | 1.1 | 1.3 | 18 | 1.5 | 1.5 | 200 | 40 | 700 | 1,000 | 11.3 | 9.5 |
| 19–50 years | 55.5 | 1.0 | 1.3 | 17 | 1.4 | 1.5 | 200 | 40 | 700 | 700 | 8.7 | 9.5 |
| 50+ years | 53.3 | 0.9 | 1.3 | 16 | 1.4 | 1.5 | 200 | 40 | 700 | 700 | 8.7 | 9.5 |

| Females | Protein (g) | Vit. B1 (mg) | Vit. B2 (mg) | Niacin (mg) | Vit. B6 (mg) | Vit. B12 (mcg) | Folate (mcg) | Vit. C (mg) | Vit. A (mcg) | Calcium (mg) | Iron (mg) | Zinc (mg) |
|---|---|---|---|---|---|---|---|---|---|---|---|---|
| 1–3 years | 14.5 | 0.5 | 0.6 | 8 | 0.7 | 0.5 | 70 | 30 | 400 | 350 | 6.9 | 5.0 |
| 4–6 years | 19.7 | 0.7 | 0.8 | 11 | 0.9 | 0.8 | 100 | 30 | 500 | 450 | 6.1 | 6.5 |
| 7–10 years | 28.3 | 0.7 | 1.0 | 12 | 1.0 | 1.0 | 150 | 30 | 500 | 550 | 8.7 | 7.0 |
| 11–14 years | 41.2 | 0.7 | 1.1 | 12 | 1.0 | 1.2 | 200 | 35 | 600 | 800 | 14.8** | 9.0 |
| 15–18 years | 45.0 | 0.8 | 1.1 | 14 | 1.2 | 1.5 | 200 | 40 | 600 | 800 | 14.8** | 7.0 |
| 19–50 years | 45.0 | 0.8 | 1.1 | 13 | 1.2 | 1.5 | 200 | 40 | 600 | 700 | 14.8** | 7.0 |
| 50+ years | 46.5 | 0.8 | 1.1 | 12 | 1.2 | 1.5 | 200 | 40 | 600 | 700 | 8.7 | 7.0 |
| Pregnancy | +6 | +0.1* | +0.3 | – | – | – | +100 | +10 | +100 | – | – | – |
| Lactation | | | | | | | | | | | | |
| 0–4 months | +11 | +0.2 | +0.5 | +2 | – | +0.5 | +60 | +30 | +350 | +550 | – | +6.0 |
| 4+ months | +8 | +0.2 | +0.5 | +2 | – | +0.5 | +60 | +30 | +350 | +550 | – | +2.5 |

– no increase
* last trimester only
** insufficient for women with high menstrual losses

From: *Dietary Reference Values for Food Energy and Nutrients for the United Kingdom*, HMSO, London (1990). Reproduced with the permission of the Controller, HMSO.

# APPENDIX 8

## Vitamins and their sources

| Vitamin | Synonym | Sources |
|---------|---------|---------|
| A | Retinol | Fish liver oil, liver, kidney, dairy produce, margarine, egg yolks, yellow and dark green vegetables |
| B1 | Thiamin | Yeast, wholemeal bread and cereals, lean pork and bacon, liver, nuts, milk, eggs, pulses and other vegetables |
| B2 | Riboflavin | Milk, liver, eggs, cheese, wholemeal bread and cereals, green vegetables |
| B3 | Niacin | Meat, fish, wholemeal bread and cereals, pulses, nuts, yeast and meat extracts |
| B6 | Pyridoxine | Liver, kidney and other meats, wholemeal cereals, nuts, seeds, bananas, fish |
| B12 | Cyanocobalamin | Liver, kidney, oily fish, eggs, cheese and milk |
|  | Folic acid | Liver, kidney, eggs, pulses, green vegetables, avocado pears, bananas, orange juice |
| C | Ascorbic acid | Citrus fruit, blackcurrants, rosehips, raw green vegetables, potatoes, tomatoes, strawberries |
| D | Calciferol | (Sunlight), oily fish, eggs, margarine, butter |
| E | Tocopherol | Wheatgerm, egg yolk, nuts, seeds and seed oils; margarines made from seed oils; green plants |

# APPENDIX 9

## Recommended weight for height

**Your height in feet and inches**
*(1 foot = approx 0.3 metres)*

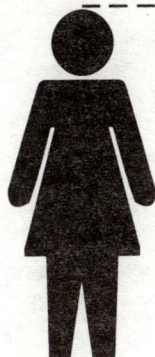

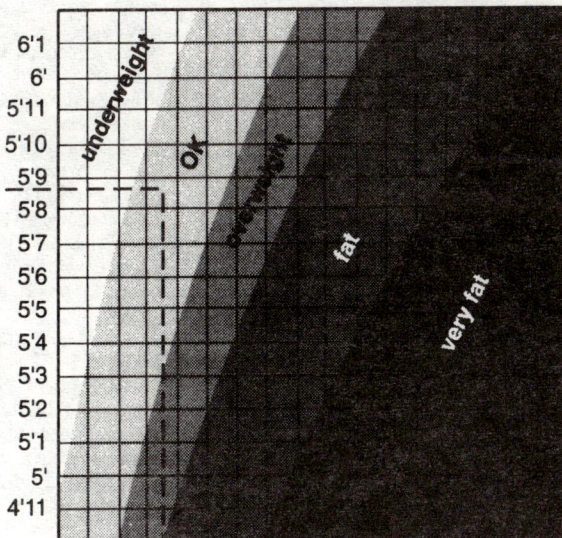

6'1
6'
5'11
5'10
5'9
5'8
5'7
5'6
5'5
5'4
5'3
5'2
5'1
5'
4'11

underweight

Ok

overweight

fat

very fat

7  8  9  10 11 12 13 14 15 16 17 18 19 20 21 22 23

**Your weight in stones** *(1 pound - approx 0.45 kilograms)*

# INDEX